Heal Your Gut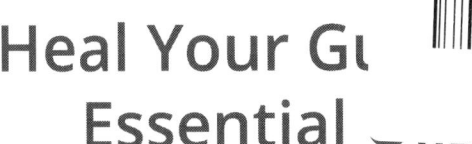
Essential...

2nd Ed (Updated & Expanded)

by Dr. Eric Zielinski

Copyright © 2019 by Biblical Health Publishing.

All rights reserved. No part of this publication may be reproduced, stored in a retrieval system, or transmitted by any means – electronic, mechanical, photographic (photocopying), recording, or otherwise – without prior permission in writing from the author.

The products and statements in this book have not been evaluated by the United States Food and Drug Administration (FDA) and are not intended to diagnose, treat, cure or prevent disease. All information provided in this book is for informational purposes only, and is not intended as a substitute for advice from your physician or other health care professional. You should not use the information in this book for diagnosis or treatment of any health problem.

Watch a FREE Screening of My 10-Part Video Masterclass to Transform Your Home (and Life!) with Essential Oils... Reserve Your Spot Today!
EssentialOilsForAbundantLiving.com

Looking for More?

Join Dr. Z's Essential Oils Club for Monthly Q & A's, Expert Interviews & More!
EssentialOilsClub.info

Other Books By Dr. Z:

The Healing Power of Essential Oils
HealingPowerOfEssentialOils.com

The Essential Oils Diet
EssentialOilsDiet.com

Table of Contents

Preface	5
Introduction	7
Section 1: Using Essential Oils Safely and Effectively	17
Chapter 1: Aromatherapy 101	18
Chapter 2: Using Carrier Oils for Double Benefits	32
Chapter 3: Ingesting Essential Oils: Are They Safe for Internal Use or Not	40
Chapter 4: Where to Buy Essential Oils and Choosing the Best Brand for You	54
Section 2: Essential Oils and Gut Health	67
Chapter 5: Maximizing Gut Health with Essential Oils	68
Chapter 6: DIY Essential Oil Protocol for Gut Health	77
Section 3: Gut Healing Essential Oil Profiles	83
Chapter 7: 5 Health Benefits of Anise Oil	84
Chapter 8: Fight Cancer and Nausea with Cardamom Essential Oil	89
Chapter 9: Cinnamon Essential Oil for Cancer, Diabetes and More	93
Chapter 10: Fennel Oil Remedy for Anxiety, Cramps and Indigestion	98
Chapter 11: Ginger Oil for Digestive Support and Cancer Prevention	106
Chapter 12: 10 Peppermint Essential Oil Uses to Live By	110
Chapter 13: Ancient Digestive Remedy: Tarragon Essential Oil	115
Chapter 14: Thyme Essential Oil Healing Power and Practical Uses	120
Conclusion	124
References	127
About the Author	135

Preface

There's a reason we shorten the Standard American Diet to S-A-D. Never has a more fitting abbreviation been seen in the health industry. Our food, and the way our body processes that food, impacts our health in profound ways.

And, it all starts in the gut.

Put simply, when our gut isn't healthy and happy, nothing about our bodies is healthy and happy. Gut health and digestive issues are one of the most common concerns shared by our Natural Living Family and most of them ask me about ways essential oils can help.

This book is a direct result of those queries, and the research I've done on the topic.

Getting the Most Out of this Book

Before you dive in, though, let me remind you that continuing a S-A-D lifestyle and using essential oils is like taking one step forward, and two steps back. The only way to truly heal the gut, regain control of your health and feel like you want to again is by taking a holistic approach.

- Diet
- Exercise
- Prayer & meditation
- Stress reduction & mood balancing
- Positive thinking & fruitful relationships
- Using natural remedies like essential oils

These are all part of the equation.

As you start your journey, my recommendation is that you first treat the symptoms related to your gut health issues. For example, using lavender to help you sleep better, or peppermint to reduce bloating. Something (anything) to get you on the road to victory! This will give you some "quick wins" and will help motivate and encourage you for the long haul. Then, once you start to feel a little better (this should happen within days of following the various protocols and recipes in this book), tackle the root cause. If you're not sure where to start, then contact a local functional medicine practitioner who understands how natural therapies like essential oils work with the body and you try to discover the "WHY" behind your health issues.

May you be blessed with an abundant life for you and your family.

~ Dr. Z

Introduction
A Starting Point with Huge Benefits

I never really had the chance to become healthy as a child because my parents were receiving misguided medical advice that led us right into a medical trap that I refer to as the *Gut Health Trifecta*:

1. Gut-Brain-Skin Axis
2. Antibiotics
3. Standard American Diet (SAD)

If the foundation isn't set, then the building will fall. It's as simple as that.

Don't discount the importance of gut health. It is responsible for up to 80% of your immune function!

Gut-Brain-Skin Axis

Gut health is intricately connected to virtually every aspect of your health. It's been nearly 80 years since dermatologists Donald M. Pillsbury and John H. Stokes first proposed the link between gut health, depression, anxiety, and skin conditions such as acne.

Known as the "Gut-Brain-Skin Axis" theory, this connection is understood to be a two-way street: emotional states can alter your normal intestinal microflora, which can increase intestinal permeability (leaky gut) and contribute to systemic inflammation. And vice versa—your microflora can influence your emotional states because these vitally important "good" bacteria produce neurotransmitters, or chemical messengers that play a role in mood and cognitive function. In my case, lacking the antibody- and probiotic-rich colostrum and breast milk in my diet as a baby, research supports my suspicion that being formula fed was the primary cause of my poor gut health.

According to the Proceedings of the *National Academy of Sciences of the United States of America,*

> *"We found that breast milk-derived SIgA [antibodies] promoted intestinal epithelial barrier function in suckling neonates, preventing systemic infection by potential pathogens. Long-term benefits of early exposure to SIgA included maintenance of a healthy gut microbiota and regulation of gene expression in intestinal epithelial cells. These findings suggest that maternal antibodies provide benefits to the intestinal immune system of the breast-fed infant, which persist into adulthood."*

Couple that with the Standard American Diet (SAD) that I consumed being low in naturally fermented foods, my poor gut health can, thus, be linked to the multitude maladies that plagued me in my youth:

- Acne
- Anxiety
- Childhood dental cavities
- Depression
- Intestinal permeability (leaky gut)
- Social phobias
- Stammering (associated with anxiety)
- Suicide ideation (associated with acne)
- Tonsillitis

The key takeaway here is that consuming a probiotic-rich diet and breastfeeding are both critical to our physical, mental and emotional health. Eating fermented foods like kimchi, sauerkraut, pickles, natto and yogurt are easy to incorporate into your health regimen. When you slip and don't to eat them for a while, that's where probiotic supplements are helpful.

Interestingly, when essential oils are taken with probiotics (beneficial bacteria in supplement form)and probiotic-rich foods they have a synergistic effect! In 2012, a study analyzing the development of a probiotic found that essential oils work well with the formula, creating a synergistic effect of increased benefits.

According to the study, *"The probiotics retard the growth of the microorganisms, while essential oil kills them. Combining the effect* of medicinal plant extract and probiotics may be a new approach due to their complementary antimicrobial effects and practically no side effects. The synergistic effect of the essential oil and probiotics will be necessarily higher than using them alone as health product."

Regarding nursing, it is important to note human breast milk is the perfect food for infants. Somehow, this minor fact has been omitted by baby formula labels. The fastest growing packaged food source to date, the global infant nutrition industry is a $50 billion market and their revenue growth is only expected to increase.

The advice that far too many moms-to-be receive—that breast milk isn't necessary and that you're putting your babies at risk of malnutrition if you decide to nurse—is simply not true.

If you're pregnant, want to be, or know someone who is, I implore you to consider these things and make a determined effort to nurse your baby for at least one full year.

For some proven tips on how to use essential oils to help you produce an ample of milk for your baby and to help ease some of the symptoms associate with baby blue that prevents some women from nursing, be sure to check out the Fennel Essential Oil chapter in this book and this article on our website, **NaturalLivingFamily.com/natural-breastfeeding-tips**.

Antibiotics

Whether intended to treat a urinary tract, strep, or staph infection, far too many antibiotics are being prescribed when essential oils could be used instead!

According to the Centers for Disease Control and Prevention, *"Up to one-third to one-half of antibiotic use in humans is either unnecessary or inappropriate. Each year in the United States, 47 million unnecessary antibiotic prescriptions are written in doctor's offices, emergency rooms, and hospital-based clinics, which makes improving antibiotic prescribing and use a national priority."*

Overuse of antibiotics has caused an outbreak of infection and is becoming a main cause of death. Each year in the United States alone, more than two million people become infected with bacteria that are resistant to antibiotics and more than 23,000 people die every year as a direct result of these infections.

If you're thinking of taking an antibiotic, consider using essential oils for all non-serious infections.

Standard American Diet

Eating processed and sugary foods every day and using essential oils is like taking one step forward and three steps back!

My challenge to you is to think, *"What would Jesus eat?"* If Christ were living on this planet today, would He eat or drink anything that could potentially cause His body harm? What do you honestly think? We cover this topic in greater detail in our book, *The Essential Oils Diet* (**EssentialOilsDiet.com**).

As we see in the Bible 2,000 years ago, Christ's life purpose was to honor God in everything that He said, thought and did; even to point of dying on the cross. Although I won't be able to prove it on this side of Heaven, I cannot logically see any way that He would have consumed anything that could possibly have hindered His ministry. And don't mistake it, everything that we eat and drink directly affects our mental, emotional, social, and physical health.

Sadly, this revelation hasn't reached mainstream Christendom. As one of my preacher friends quipped, "Christians don't drink, they don't smoke, they eat!" An argument can be made that gluttony is the acceptable sin in the church. Or, at least it appears this way because I don't hear too many ministers preaching against it!

I have seen the lives of far too many pastors, missionaries, and church leaders cut short because of disease; many of which could have all but been prevented by lifestyle changes. This, my friend, is the antithesis of Biblical health: seeing spiritual "giants" fall apart at the hands of poor lifestyle decisions.

The remedies presented in this book presuppose that you're adopting healthy diet, fitness, and lifestyle habits that necessitate healing.

A Note About Faith

As I shard, my personal health journey has included gut issues since as far as I can remember and I credit God for showing me how to heal myself from the inside-out.

Jehovah Rapha: The Lord, Our Healer. There are dozens of Bible verses about healing and I have come to take solace in these over the years as my loved ones and I have battle health conditions. They have brought up comfort, hope and have built up our most holy faith to believe our Lord for a miracle!

With that said, there is a practical application to all of this. The Lord has gifted your body with the remarkable ability to heal itself under the right conditions. You need to feed it wholesome food, drink clean water and breathe pure air.

Sadly, finding these things is all but impossible in our fallen world as toxic chemicals have overtaken our soil and atmosphere. In spite of our efforts (and great expense) to purchase essential products for a healthy home, we still get sick and God is here to bless you with His healing touch when you need it. My prayer is that you find this precious gift, and these Healing Scriptures encourage you along the way!

Old Testament Healing Scriptures

He said, "If you will diligently listen to the voice of the Lord your God, and do that which is right in his eyes, and give ear to his commandments and keep all his statutes, I will put none of the diseases on you that I put on the Egyptians, for I am the Lord, your healer."
~ **Exodus 15:26**

Worship the LORD your God, and His blessing will be on your food and water. I will take away sickness from among you.
~ **Exodus 23:25**

The Lord will keep you free from every disease. He will not inflict on you the horrible diseases you knew in Egypt.
~ **Deuteronomy 7:15**

See now that I, even I, am he, and there is no god beside me; I kill and I make alive; I wound and I heal; and there is none that can deliver out of my hand.
~ **Deuteronomy 32:39**

If my people who are called by my name humble themselves, and pray and seek my face and turn from their wicked ways, then I will hear from heaven and will forgive their sin and heal their land.
~ **2 Chronicles 7:14**

Have compassion on me, LORD, for I am weak. Heal me, LORD, for my bones are in agony.
~ **Psalm 6:2**

For the LORD protects the bones of the righteous; not one of them is broken!
~ **Psalm 34:20**

The LORD will sustain him upon his sickbed; In his illness, You restore him to health.
~ **Psalm 41:3**

As for me, I said, "O Lord, be gracious to me; heal me, for I have sinned against you!"
~ **Psalm 41:4**

Praise the Lord, my soul; all my inmost being, praise his holy name. Praise the Lord, my soul, and forget not all his benefits—who forgives all your sins and heals all your diseases, who redeems your life from the pit and crowns you with love and compassion, who satisfies your desires with good thing, so that your youth is renewed like the eagle's.
~ **Psalm 103:1-5**

He sent out His word and healed them, and delivered them from their destruction.
~ **Psalm 107:20**

He heals the brokenhearted and binds up their wounds.
~ **Psalm 147:3**

Gracious words are like a honeycomb, sweetness to the soul and health to the body.
~ **Proverbs 16:24**

My son, be attentive to my words; incline your ear to my sayings. Let them not escape from your sight; keep them within your heart. For they are life to those who find them, and healing to all their flesh.
~ **Proverbs 4:20-22**

A joyful heart is good medicine, but a crushed spirit dries up the bones.
~ **Proverbs 17:22**

For everything there is a season, and a time for every matter under heaven: a time to be born, and a time to die; a time to plant, and a time to pluck up what is planted; a time to kill, and a time to heal; a time to break down, and a time to build up.
~ **Ecclesiastes 3:1-3**

And the Lord will strike Egypt, striking and healing, and they will return to the Lord, and he will listen to their pleas for mercy and heal them.
~ **Isaiah 19:22**

Lord, your discipline is good, for it leads to life and health. You restore my health and allow me to live!
~ **Isaiah 38:16**

But He was pierced for our transgressions, He was crushed for our iniquities; the punishment that brought us peace was on Him, and by His wounds we are healed.
~ **Isaiah 53:5**

'I have seen what they do, but I will heal them anyway! I will lead them. I will comfort those who mourn, bringing words of praise to their lips. May they have abundant peace, both near and far,' says the Lord, who heals them.
~ **Isaiah 57: 18-19**

Then your light will break forth like the dawn, and your healing will quickly appear; then your righteousness will go before you, and the glory of the LORD will be your rear guard.

~ **Isaiah 58:8**

Heal me, O Lord, and I shall be healed; save me, and I shall be saved, for you are my praise.

~ **Jeremiah 17:14**

For I will restore health to you, and your wounds I will heal, declares the Lord.

~ **Jeremiah 30:17**

Behold, I will bring to it health and healing, and I will heal them and reveal to them abundance of prosperity and security.

~ **Jeremiah 33:6**

New Testament Healing Scriptures

And he went throughout all Galilee, teaching in their synagogues and proclaiming the gospel of the kingdom and healing every disease and every affliction among the people.

~ **Matthew 4:23**

And He called to Him His twelve disciples and gave them authority over unclean spirits, to cast them out, and to heal every disease and every affliction.

~ **Matthew 10:1**

Heal the sick, raise the dead, cleanse those who have leprosy, drive out demons. Freely you have received; freely give.

~ **Matthew 10:8**

It is not the healthy who need a doctor, but the sick. I have not come to call the righteous, but sinners.

~ **Mark 2:17**

He [Jesus] said to her, "Daughter, your faith has healed you. Go in peace and be freed from your suffering."

~ **Mark 5:34**

And the power of the Lord was with him to heal.

~ **Luke 5:17**

Heal the sick in it and say to them, 'The kingdom of God has come near to you.'

~ **Luke 10:9**

And He laid His hands on her, and immediately she was made straight, and she glorified God.

~ **Luke 13:13**

But they remained silent. Then He took him and healed him and sent him away.

~ **Luke 14:4**

"He has blinded their eyes and hardened their heart, lest they see with their eyes, and understand with their heart, and turn, and I would heal them."

~ **John 12:40**

While you stretch out your hand to heal, and signs and wonders are performed through the name of your holy servant Jesus.

~ **Acts 4:30**

And Peter said to him, "Aeneas, Jesus Christ heals you; rise and make your bed." And immediately he rose.

~ **Acts 9:34**

How God anointed Jesus of Nazareth with the Holy Spirit and with power. He went about doing good and healing all who were oppressed by the devil, for God was with him.

~ **Acts 10:38**

Our bodies are buried in brokenness, but they will be raised in glory. They are buried in weakness, but they will be raised in strength.

~ **1 Corinthians 15:43**

Is anyone among you sick? Let him call for the elders of the church, and let them pray over him, anointing him with oil in the name of the Lord. And the prayer of faith will save the one who is sick, and the Lord will raise him up.

~ James 5:14-15

Therefore, confess your sins to one another and pray for one another, that you may be healed. The effectual fervent prayer of a righteous man availeth much.

~ James 5:16

He personally bore our sins in His [own] body on the tree [as on an altar and offered Himself on it], that we might die (cease to exist) to sin and live to righteousness. By His wounds you have been healed.

~ 1 Peter 2:24

Dear friend, I pray that you may enjoy good health and that all may go well with you, even as your soul is getting along well.

~ 3 John 1:2

Which of these 40 Bible verses about healing Scriptures speaks to your heart?

Send me an email at **Support@NaturalLivingFamily.com** and let me know!

Section 1

Using Essential Oils Safely and Effectively

Chapter 1
Aromatherapy 101: Guide to Safe and Effective Use

Although the use of essential oils isn't new, it has definitely gained a wild fanfare in recent years. More and more people are using essential oils in place of artificial fragrances in the home and on their bodies, for culinary purposes, and for health and healing. The more we use essential oils, the more we fall in love, and it's hard to remember a time when aromatherapy was an unfamiliar term.

Everyone has to start somewhere, though – few of us were born into families who already used essential oils regularly. If you are just starting out and find yourself a bit lost in the jargon, recipes, and excitement, don't worry. You aren't alone. Let's take a little bit of time here and catch you up to speed.

Our Favorite Essential Oils Blends

I'm not sure about you, but my wife and I utilize essential oils all day long. It enhances our mood, health and virtually every aspect of our lives! We have an essential oil diffuser in nearly every room in our home, and once we gave all those toxic plug-ins and aerosols the boot, we started to notice some pretty cool changes in our health and the health of our children.

These are some of our favorite blends (1:1:1:1 ratio):

- **Goodbye Allergy Blend** – Lavender, lemon, and peppermint
- **Healthy Digestion Blend** – Anise, caraway, fennel, ginger, lemon, tarragon
- **Focus Blend** – Cedarwood, frankincense, sandalwood and vetiver
- **Christmas Blend** – Fir (Balsam, Douglas, white), peppermint and vanilla absolute
- **Holy Anointing Blend** – cinnamon, frankincense, myrrh

- **Immune Boosting Blend** – Cinnamon, clove, eucalyptus, rosemary, orange and lemon
- **Joyful Blend** – Orange, lemon, bergamot, grapefruit and vanilla absolute
- **Deep Breathing Blend** – Cardamom, eucalyptus, lemon, peppermint, rosemary, tea tree
- **Sleepy Time Blend** – Roman chamomile, lavender, and vetiver

At this point, you may be asking, *"How can these aromatherapy blends make a difference in my life?"*

Well, it's all about the healing power of essential oils...

What are Essential Oils?

"And the leaves of the tree are for the healing of the nations." (Revelation 22:2)

I can think of no other substance on earth that epitomizes this Bible verse than essential oils.

The very first questions a newbie should ask – what is aromatherapy, and what is an essential oil? You might associate aromatherapy with massage therapists and thick massage oil. Or perhaps you picture heavy patchouli incense and a Volkswagen van. Or the base, middle, and high notes of a perfumery concoctions.

All of these can be accurate associations with aromatherapy – while at the same time, each of them may or may not be using essential oils.

The term *essential* oil doesn't refer to how much we need it (though many of us argue that they are pretty vital parts of our daily lives!). In fact, the original scientific term for these oils is *volatile oil,* which paints a much better picture of what we're referring to.

The volatile oil – or essential oil – of a plant is the part that releases quickly from the plant and into the air. The *Encyclopedia Britannica* describes the naming rationale:

"Essential oil, highly volatile substance isolated by a physical process from an odoriferous plant of a single botanical species...Such oils were called essential because they were thought to represent the very essence of odor and flavor."

The essential oil is why you smell a rose when you lean down and sniff the blooms. It releases as you walk through the garden and shake up the plants. How many plants can you identify by their scent alone? The scientists who had the privilege of naming this chemical component could think of plenty, as well, and thus believed the oils to be "essential" to the plant as much as it was volatile (quickly released).

We now know that essential oils are more prevalent in some plants than others, and can be found in roots, stems, leaves, and blossoms alike. They aren't necessarily an essential part of the plant – in fact, we don't always know the function the volatile oil serves, and it can very from plant to plant. But we do know that essential oils are complex, with broad therapeutic actions that vary based on their composition.

Ultimately, the essential oil of a plant is a component of the plant itself, filled with vast amounts of molecules specific to that plant's needs and uses. This is important to remember, because chemical composition (*phytochemistry*, the chemistry of plants), tells us how we can best use a substance.

History of Aromatherapy

More recently, essential oils have been used under the guise of the aromatherapy profession, although we have records of people using them as far as thousands of years ago. Did they have essential oils like we know them today? Of course not! Modern distillation procedures are relatively new in relation to the Earth timetable. However, Nicander (b.c. 183—135), a Greek poet and physician for example, "Spoke of the extraction of perfumes from plants by what we should now call a process of distillation" and we have other ancient accounts of crude methods to extract the precious oil from plants.

The term *aromatherapy* is relatively new in our history, coined by a French chemist named Rene-Maurice Gattefosse in the 1930s. His work ultimately led to the modern understanding of essential oils as therapeutic for health and healing benefits.

This shift toward isolating and emphasizing the use of essential oils as a separate and concentrated compounds with the goal of therapeutic results has shaped what we know about essential oils today. It gave us the vials of pure essential oils, separate from the other compounds they shared space with in the larger composition of a plant. But it wasn't the first time essential oils were recognized for their healing abilities.

Because essential oils are part of herbs – the aromatic compound that hits your nose right away – they can be part of herbal preparations. The practice of using herbs as medicine dates back to the beginning of human history, and since we have always had noses, the fragrant component of those herbs did not go unnoticed.

Most civilizations utilized fragrant herbs for medicine and rituals, and oil extractions were commonly used to separate the fragrance and medicinal benefits from the bulkier material of the rest of the plant. Many of the oils used in this way were rich in essential oils that we continue to use to this day – myrrh, cinnamon, frankincense, cassia – prized for their fragrances and traded vigorously throughout the ancient world and into the development of the Western world we know today.

The 'spices' were burned, infused into carrier oils, and even crudely distilled. This crude distillation produced something similar to what we nowadays call hydrosols, which contain minute amounts of the essential oil from the distillation process.

Today, thanks to pioneers such as Gattefosse, we really do have essential oil extraction down to a science, and we're learning more all the time.

Herbal Preparations vs. Essential Oils

There is no doubt that the ancients realized the fragrance was something more than just pleasant. Such was the confidence in the therapeutic power of aromas that, at one point, the entire prevailing theory of disease centered around bad and good smells!

So when we talk about essential oils being used from ancient times – for example, in the Bible, when fragrant offerings were commanded and incense was to be burned – it's true in that the essential oils were present and utilizing the fragrance was the intended result.

Where ancient and modern use differs, however, is that we are now able to isolate the essential oil – not simply include it, but use it exclusively. An herbal oil is herbal matter infused with an oil such as olive, so that it contains the essential oil (albeit in very small amounts) alongside many other compounds from the plant. There are fewer compounds, obviously, since the plant matter is strained away and discarded, but there are still many, creating a highly usable oil infused with a range of medicinal properties.

The essential oils as we know them, on the other hand, take the small amount of volatile oil from part of a plant and concentrate it so that it's the only product of the plant remaining. This is usually accomplished using steam distillation to release the droplets and then catch them. Because it's an "extraction" of a very small facet of a plant, it takes large volumes of each plant to create even a 5ml bottle of essential oil.

It comes down to this: for herbed oils, the oil is now medicinally stronger than it was before, but the herbal matter is more varied and less concentrated than an essential oil.

For essential oils, the oil is concentrated and specific in use, condensed from large amounts of herbal matter that have been isolated for a single component, therefore compressed into much, much smaller volumes of oil.

To break it down further, the herbal oil can contain the essential oil but not vice versa.

How Essential Oils Work

Let's put this into practical terms. Cinnamon, for example, is a delicious spice. The cinnamon that you sprinkle onto toast is essentially ground-up bark and is the culmination of a combination of many chemical components – yes, including essential oils.

In cinnamon sticks or ground cinnamon, the oils are dispersed amongst the other components, giving you a wide range of substances to stir into tea or add to Christmas pie.

Now, to make cinnamon essential oil, that same bark would be placed through a distillation process, releasing and separating the essential oil. Great amounts of bark would be used in the process, and precious vials of essential oil would be the result.

Same bark, same plant. But would you shake your cinnamon essential oil bottle all over your morning toast, just like you did with the powder?

Putting Oils in Context of the Plant

When the essential oil – whatever is left after processing, packaging, and then your cooking methods – is part of the whole product, it is in such small and dispersed amounts that it's only a small contribution to the whole. You're enjoying powdered cinnamon for the combination of molecules that create texture, flavor, and varied benefits.

When you use an essential oil, you should use it for the very specific benefits that those specific molecules can provide. In the case of cinnamon bark, it's pretty potent as an antibacterial, more so than a dessert seasoning.

And while it still does taste great and could be used with proper care in a culinary setting (we'll get to that in a minute), it's also a dermal irritant. In other words, it could really hurt your skin or the tender lining of your mouth and throat if you were to use it just like cinnamon sticks or powder.

To throw another wrench in the works, the essential oil gathered from the bark won't have the same components as that of the essential oil taken from leaves. And it will vary between varieties of the same plant species, growing methods, seasons, and even the way it's harvested. These are *volatile* oils, remember? They are pretty delicate in their composition and will adapt based on their conditions and use to the plant.

Pretty powerful stuff! The progress that we have made since *Aromatherapie* was first written allows us to choose essential oils for specific uses based on what we know of their composition. Rather than burning whatever smells good and hoping it chases away disease, we can combine the art and science of aromatherapy to be intentional and effective in our use.

How Essential Oils are Used

The term *aromatherapy* was coined to combine aroma and therapy, indicating therapeutic benefits using fragrance. This is still the heart of aromatherapy, but essential oil use has expanded in many ways and toward many uses.

The main categories of use are:
- Inhalation
- Topical
- Internal

INHALATION

Not only is inhalation the oldest form of essential oil use, it is also arguably the safest. Oils diffused throughout a room are relatively safe for most people in most cases due to the low level of concentration when used correctly.

More direct effects can be obtained by breathing in a steam directly or inhaling right from the bottle, or from a few drops on a cloth. This carries the volatile oil directly into your respiratory system and mucous membranes, diffused throughout the steam or air molecules.

TOPICAL

Topical use is a step further than traditional inhalation-based aromatherapy, though still familiar in the context of massage therapy, which often utilizes fragrant essential oils for massage applications.

Instead of the broad diffusion through air droplets that inhalation provides, topical use of essential oils is much more direct. But at the same time, the oil is absorbed through the barrier layers of skin, while inhalation moves quickly through the thinner mucous membranes. Knowing your oil and the goal you have in mind can help you determine which application is more appropriate.

In theory and in professional practice, some essential oils can be used on the skin undiluted. However, the safest application is via dilution. Carrier oils like olive, coconut, jojoba and avocado oils usually have benefits of their own, and you can easily combine a couple of drops in a teaspoon to dilute the oils and help bypass potential irritation.

INTERNAL

Finally, and most controversially, some oils are safe for ingestion. The most basic form of ingestion is in culinary use. Revisiting cinnamon, you could use cinnamon essential oil in a cake batter, but you'd only need one drop for the whole batch vs. a tsp or more of the bark powder.

Another common internal preparation is to combine it into a drink. Do remember that oil and water *do not mix*, so simply adding a drop to water will leave that drop undiluted. Some oils are irritants and all oils are very strong, so it's best to be safe and dilute it into some coconut oil first.

Many aromatherapists believe essential oils are never to be ingested, and most will suggest only trained professionals utilize internal methods. Again, it's better to be safe, and for someone just starting out, this is excellent advice to consider. Additionally, when you are dealing with a specific medical condition, it makes sense to talk to your health care provider about ingestion and dosages.

Conversions and Dilution of Essential Oils

Dropper sizes vary and volume varies based on oil, so advanced techniques would include more specific measuring techniques. Most bottles that I've seen contain either 5 ml or 15 ml of oil, which would be 100 drops or 300 drops, respectively. For you math enthusiasts out there, this is how the conversions all pan out:

- 1/8 oz. = 3.75 ml
- 1/4 oz. = 7.5 ml
- 1/2 oz. = 15 ml.
- 1 oz. = 30 ml
- 4 oz. = 120 ml
- 8 oz. = 237 ml
- 16 oz. = 473 ml

The final conversion typically looks like this:

- 1/8 oz. = 75 drops
- 1/4 oz. = 150 drops
- 1/2 oz. = 300 drops
- 1 oz. = 600 drops

Using these conversions:

- 1% dilution: 6 drops of EO per oz of carrier oil (1% of 600 drops is 6)
- 2% dilution: 12 drops of EO per oz of carrier oil (2% of 600 drops is 12)
- 3% dilution: 18 drops of EO per oz of carrier oil (3% of 600 drops is 18)

If working with tablespoons are more comfortable for you, 1 oz. = 2 tablespoons. So, there are 300 drops of EO in a tablespoon.

- 1% dilution: 3 drops of EO per tablespoon of carrier oil (1% of 300 drops is 3)
- 2% dilution: 6 drops of EO per tablespoon of carrier oil (2% of 300 drops is 6)
- 3% dilution: 9 drops of EO per tablespoon of carrier oil (3% of 300 drops is 9)

If working with grams, 1 drop of essential oil = 0.02 to 0.03 grams approximately (depending on your dropper), which converts to 20-30 milligrams or 20000 micrograms (µg).

So 30 mg is about 1 drop.

Application Methods of Essential Oils

Within the major types of essential oil use, there are many ways to actually apply them. These suggestions and guidelines can get you rolling, but once you are familiar with your oils and their safe use, you can really start to think outside of the box.

INHALATION

For inhaled oils, you only need a small amount to create a big impact. Diffusers will use a bit more, but direct inhalation is up close and personal and only requires a couple of drops. Here are some of the methods you might use to inhale essential oils.

- **Diffusion** – Good for blends intended to affect the entire room. Place as few as 2-3 and as many as 6-10 total drops in the diffuser or in a pot of simmering water and let it disperse throughout the room. It depends on the size of the water tank so be sure to follow instructions. The benefits should be lasting after the diffusion has ended; there is no need to run it continuously. *Ideally for essential oils that are energizing, antimicrobial, promoting memory and focus, relaxing. Ex: citrus, lavender, rosemary.*

- **Personal inhalation** – Good for portable, direct inhalation for specific benefits to an individual. Fewer drops are needed due to the close proximity of use. Up to 20 drops of an essential oil blend can be used in a commercially made personal inhaler. Or consider jewelry style inhalers such as a piece of porous jewelry, a piece of cloth or handkerchief, or inhalers made of a wick of sorts placed in a glass tube. Place 1-2 drops of a single oil or a pre-prepared blend of oils on the jewelry inhaler, then hold it close to the nose and breathe in periodically. *Ideally for personal benefit such as clear breathing, focus, anxiety, headaches, and stress relief. Ex: eucalyptus, bergamot, peppermint.*

- **Steam inhalation** – Technically also personal inhalation, "tenting" is more intensive and not very portable. When the essential oils need to be inhaled in greater concentration and affect the respiratory system more directly, 2-3 drops of a single oil or pre-

prepared blend can be placed in a bowl of boiling water – usually warmed in and poured from a tea kettle. Place a towel over your head and drape it over the bowl (forming a tent, of sorts), close your eyes, and breathe deeply. Avoid the more hot oils that would irritate mucous membranes. *Ideal for clearing the nasal passages and respiratory system. Ex: eucalyptus, citrus, tea tree.*

- **Sprays** – Aromatic sprays have benefits of both inhalation and, in the case of antimicrobial oils, surface cleaning benefits. Combine 10-20 drops of a combination of oils to ½ oz 190 proof grain alcohol or the 91% isopropyl you can find in the store , then add ½ oz distilled water and shake to combine. Spritz in the air, on linens, or on clothes as desired. *Ideally for air freshening, cleaning, antimicrobial purposes, body sprays, and even topical anti-inflammatory benefits and healing. Ex: tea tree, lemon, thyme.*

TOPICAL APPLICATION

Essential oils placed directly on the skin are able to sink in through the pores and then move through the body, creating both topical benefits as well as systemic. While there is a time and a place for neat application, the smart way to apply oils topically is to first dilute them. Carrier oils are non-volatile oils and are not irritants, so essential oils can be blended into them first and then the mixture applied.

Popular carrier oils include: coconut, olive, almond, jojoba, avocado, apricot, and sunflower. Most carrier oils have benefits of their own that can be explored to create even more beneficial blends.

Topical application can be direct in a small area such as for scar healing or broader such as for a massage oil. The important variables here are dilution rates.

- **0.5% dilution** – Strong oils, application on children, and oils that you are testing for sensitization. The heavy dilution allows for greater distribution throughout the application and less per dose. *Ideal for irritating oils, children, and those who are highly sensitive. Ex: cinnamon, eucalyptus, peppermint.*

- **1% dilution** – Even adults who tolerate oils well will still find some oils too strong for normal applications. A 1% dilution rate protects your skin while still enjoying the benefit of the more powerful essential oils or use on sensitive areas of the skin. *Ideal for facial applications, and treatment of delicate skin. Ex: tea tree for acne, frankincense in a facial toner, etc.*

- **2-3% dilution** – This is the most common dilution range, suitable for massage oils, healing treatments, lotions and creams, and cosmetic applications. It is enough to gain significant benefits of the essential oil without risking sensitization. Unless the oil is particularly potent or you have sensitive skin, this is likely to be the dilution you'll use. *Ideal for most applications – lotions, creams, salves, balms. Ex: geranium, helichrysum, chamomile.*

- **5%+ dilution** – Higher concentrations should be used with care. Or, extremely safe oils can be used in small amounts on small areas of the skin – for example, as a strong acne treatment. Know your oil's safety profile and choose high concentrations with caution. *Ideal for specific situations based on either extreme safety and high potency in a targeted area OR further dilution beyond the initial formula. Ex: lavender, sweet orange, tea tree.*

INGESTION

Typically reserved for culinary oils or for use by trained aromatherapy professionals, ingestion is used when there is a need for specific dosing or certain areas of the body need to be reached that cannot easily be affected by other application methods. Dosage is important, as does education before use. Some of the more common ways ingestion is used are highlighted here.

- Excellent for digestive oils or simply to enjoy the flavorful concentration, 1-2 drops can be mixed thoroughly into a lipid or syrup portion of the recipe and then added to the rest of the batch. *Ideal for oils that benefit digestive wellness, essential oils of culinary herbs, and oils of culinary spices. Ex: dill, sweet orange, cinnamon.*

- Dispersing an oil into a glass of water is the quickest way to ingest it, but do not miss the importance of both dosage and dilution. One drop is more than sufficient, and remember that oil and water do not mix! Without dilution or dispersion, the drop is likely to make direct contact with sensitive internal organs. You can use a dispersing agent like Solubol for essential oils taken in water, or you can quickly mix a drop into a teaspoon of honey and take the spoonful. *Ideal for quick and simple use, especially for digestive wellness. Ex: chamomile, ginger, lavender.*

- A truly medicinal application, encapsulated oils are used to get the oil directly to the stomach, or – in the case of enteric-coated capsules – to the intestines. This is used when the oil is to be consumed regularly and when the individual struggles with the taste of it in other forms. Dilute the essential oil into a carrier before making the capsules, or purchase encapsulated oil blends already made. *Ideal for professional guidance, digestive health, and oils that need to make it directly to the intestines. Ex: peppermint, lavender, lemon.*

Beginners Guide to Essential Oils

So now that you know what an essential oil is to a plant, how to differentiate between an herbal oil and an essential oil, how the ancients used oils and how that has evolved over time to the modern science of aromatherapy – are you hooked yet?!

Aromatherapy is absolutely incredible. Plants are literally throwing these substances at us (Really! Pay attention the next time you walk past a lavender shrub). And then chemists can isolate those substances and analyze their very molecules. And THEN we can begin to study how these things impact our health? Amazing. If you aren't hooked yet, you will be once you get started.

5 Steps to Get Started with Essential Oils

1. The best place to begin with essential oils is with familiar scents. Lavender is both a familiar scent and a versatile and safe essential oil. The citrus oils are also easy to use on their own or in blends. Choose a few, and then learn all you can about them.

2. Next, locate a source and make your purchase. Remember that it takes large amounts of plant matter to make small amounts of oil, so a cheap bottle of a precious oil is not likely to be high quality. You want real essential oils – nothing synthetic – and always pure, especially if you are going to learn to safely ingest them.

3. Once you have a few oils ready to go, start by diffusing them on their own, and then in combinations of a couple of drops of two or three of them at a time. You can buy a diffuser, or you can simply simmer a pot of water on the stove and add your drops there.

4. When you are familiar and comfortable with the scents, you will start to learn what blends you like. As you learn more about their effects, you can begin to create blends for specific reasons, like energizing your sluggish afternoon or clearing the air after a virus passed through the house.

5. From there, you can begin to experiment with diluted topical applications, like a soothing peppermint rub or a calming massage.

The important thing is to always be learning – never stop learning! The more we learn and grow, the better we can utilize these precious, truly essential oils.

Chapter 2
Using Carrier Oils for Double Benefits

When reading about essential oils – whether you are brand new to essential oils or digging for new recipe blends – you'll often see a carrier or base oil included in the discussion, or see mention of dilution. So what is a carrier oil, and how do you know which carrier oils to get?

The carrier oil is a fatty extract, usually cold pressed from its source. Individual allergies aside, carrier oils are not likely to cause sensitization and therefore make an excellent medium to disperse the more concentrated essential oil across your skin.

Carrier oils are nutritive and have healing properties of their own, so in your discovery of essential oils, don't forget to take some time to learn about your options for carrier oils, as well.

When to Use Carrier Oils

Before you ask – yes, carrier oils are necessary! Once you get the hang of it, adding your essential oils to a carrier first is hardly any extra work, and in return you are actually amplifying the efficacy of your healing application.

It might seem backwards to say that diluting a substance makes it more effective, but in this case it is true. Essential oil applications without carrier oils (called "neat" applications) put the oil directly onto your skin. A few things of note are happening here:

1. The skin may be sensitized to the concentrated oil, harming the body by creating an allergic response.

2. The essential oil may quickly evaporate off the surface of the skin, whereas the lipids in a carrier can help drive it into the pores. Remember, essential oils are "volatile organic compounds," which means that they are emitted as gas when

exposed to open air. This is why you may notice their aroma within seconds of opening the bottle.

3. You can't massage it in or disperse it across wider spaces.

4. An ingested neat oil may cling to the mucous membranes and never make it to the intended site of application.

5. Not to mention, ingesting neat oils can easily burn your mouth and irritate your esophagus!

Bottom line: using essential oils undiluted is largely a waste of time, money and can place your body in harm's way. While there are instances when neat is acceptable – gentle oils, or oils under the supervision of a trained aromatherapist – your best bet is to dilute essential oils into a carrier every time.

Without essential oils, you will also use carriers as the base of most DIY herbal preparations, from lotion bars to chapstick to salves. Start with the most accessible carrier oils, then work through others as you learn their benefits and ideal uses.

4 Categories of Carrier Oils to Know

Herbal supply stores, health food stores, and online supply shops will offer you dozens of carrier oils to choose from. Don't get overwhelmed at your options! What is a carrier oil? Carrier oils are relatively simple to understand, and for most preparations, you can't really go wrong.

We'll walk through the more common of the carrier oils here, but if you run into one you aren't sure about that isn't covered here, take the time to look it up and learn what it is and does. Self-education may not teach us everything, but it can take us a long way if we pursue it.

1. BEGINNER CARRIER OILS: OLIVE AND COCONUT

The best place to start is at the beginning, and for DIY aromatic and herbal preparations, that's right in your own kitchen. Really, if we take it back to Hippocrates encouraging us to find our medicine in our food, the kitchen has been the starting point for many generations!

Let's spend a bit of time on these two, as this is likely where you'll start with carrier oils and diluted topical preparations before branching out to other carrier oils.

Olive Oil – Almost undoubtedly in your kitchen, as it is probably the most commonly used culinary and carrier oil out there. Because it is used so much, however, it may be adulterated with similarly-colored sunflower and corn oils. Once again, we are reminded to check our product sources carefully! Extra virgin olive oil – which is cold pressed and minimally processed – is the ideal, and it will be a light green color with a thick scent.

Sometimes, the scent can be off-putting, so you'll want to choose olive oil when making a highly aromatic blend or preparation. In 2015, a double-blind, randomized study took place in which olive oil was used on diabetic patients with ulcers on their feet. After four weeks of treatment, the patients who'd received olive oil topical treatments had smaller, less pronounced ulcers than those who received placebo or nothing. The use of olive oil as a carrier can add to the soothing, healing effects of your dilutions and preparations.

Choose this when: Making homemade salves, creams and oil pulling. Good for dry skin.

Coconut Oil – A saturated fat taken from coconuts, which are actually giant seeds. The oil drives into the skin easily with very little greasy residue, taking the oils you've blended in with it. Even without anything blended into it, coconut oil has been shown to enhance the wound healing process. You probably already use coconut oil regularly; its popularity has recently sparked internet jokes about how much you can do with coconut oil: fix your hair, fix your budget, fix your significant other...The jokes, of course are rooted in reality, poking good-natured fun at the almost comical range of things you can do with coconut oil.

Choose this when: Making most of your DIY projects and is a nice massage oil carrier. Tasty addition to your oil pulling ritual. And is best for dry skin as it leaves a little oily residue.

The way coconut oil is processed will affect its uses. Cold pressed coconut oil (virgin, extra virgin) will retain the coconut scent and will become solid when room temperature or cooler. Heat processed coconut oil will not have the taste and smell of coconut, and fractionated coconut oil (the most processed of the options) will not become solid. The tendency to solidify can be good or bad for your preparations – for quick dilutions, it is sometimes nice to mix up the essential oil into a semi-solid coconut oil and then be able to rub on a quick-melting preparation as it warms to your skin.

Fractionated Coconut Oil – Literally a fraction of the coconut oil – being that all of the long chain triglycerides have been removed – fractionated coconut oil is a lightweight emollient that is a must-have for dry or sensitive skin. Also referred to as FCO, It provides an effective barrier without clogging pores and leaves your skin feeling smooth and never greasy.

FCO is considered to be the most cost-effective oil because it will never go rancid, and helps preserve the shelf life of your essential oils if blended. In fact, some suppliers claim that it can be mixed with other (more expensive) carrier oils to extend their shelf life. It is colorless and odorless, and it incorporates perfectly with other oils without altering their scent, appearance or effectiveness.

Chose this when: Quick dilutions with what you have on hand; enhancing skin healing; perfect to treat health conditions like infections, open wounds and chronic disease.

2. NUT & SEED CARRIER OILS: ALMOND AND JOJOBA

These oils are probably not in your kitchen for cooking, but they are still very commonly purchased, easy to work with, and rich sources of skin-health nutrients. If you are ready to take a step beyond your pantry, these make a good place to start.

Almond Oil – Very mild in scent and flavor, almond oil is nutrient dense and versatile. Almond oil is a good topical source vitamins A & E, adding to the many nutritional benefits that almonds have simply as a food. Traditional uses indicate almond oil for dry skin conditions, like psoriasis and eczema, and its nutrient level and ability to penetrate the skin seems to support this use. As an emollient, almond oil can be soothing for sore skin.

Jojoba Oil – If you've not yet heard of jojoba (or heard it pronounced), it's *ho-HO-ba* that you are looking for. Derived from the seeds, jojoba is actually classified as a liquid wax, which adds another layer to your carrier oil choice. It doesn't solidify as quickly as coconut oil does, but the consistency is well suited to deep penetration and moisturizing. Jojoba has an excellent shelf life, which is perfect for storing until you need it for small dilution preparations. It has been studied for anti-inflammatory properties, wound healing ability, and efficacy in face-mask treatments for acne. It's one of Sabrina's favorite and she uses it as a base for her carrier oil blend.

Choose these when: Skin is dry or inflamed; nutrients are lacking; versatility and ease of use are desired. Good for most DIY projects.

Rosehip Seed Oil – This is one of Sabrina's favorite carrier oils for skin conditions. You don't have to use it solo, but it can be a great oil to add into any blend you're using to boost the nourishing richness. It's high in Vitamin C and is a soothing emollient for a variety of skin conditions. It can even be part of a skin conditioning lotion bar!

Choose this when: Whenever you need additional support for your skin or add this into healing skin serum.

3. FRUIT CARRIER OILS: APRICOT, AVOCADO, AND GRAPESEED

Easy to remember thanks to kitchen staples, these oils typically come from the seeds of their respective fruits, as is the case with the other carrier oils. These choices are as affordable and accessible as they are versatile.

Apricot Oil – Available as expeller pressed or cold pressed, the difference is simply texture and preference. Apricot oil's nutrient profile includes vitamins E and A as well, or at least the carotenoid precursor to vitamin A. It is edible as well as beneficial topically. Because it is so incredibly gentle as well as nourishing, apricot oil is a good choice for applications that will cover a good deal of skin or that will be applied on children heavily.

Avocado Oil – Avocado as a fruit is one of the best sources of fat and nutrients (and dip!) you can find. The oil itself, as you might imagine, is an emollient, taken from the smooth flesh around the pit. An exception to the typical seed-derived oil, avocado oil is rich in nutrients and excellent at penetrating the skin. In another animal trial, this one occurring in 2008, avocado oil was also found to have good wound healing ability. Before elaborating on the study, the researchers noted that the oil is *"rich in nutrient waxes, proteins and minerals, as well as vitamins A, D and E...an excellent source of enrichment for dry, damaged or chapped skin."*

Grape Seed Oil – Also a culinary oil, grape seed oil topically is used for its light texture and lack of residue. Once on and in the skin, grape seed is another oil verified for its contributions in wound care and healing. The high levels of fatty acid content and antioxidants in grape seed oil contribute to much of its beneficial composition. Without the heaviness of more saturated oils, grape seed makes a cleaner topical application with less of a greasy film.

Choose these when: Creating a massage oil; looking for deep hydration; creating chapsticks and balms.

4. ESSENTIAL FATTY ACID CARRIER OILS: BORAGE AND EVENING PRIMROSE

While most of the carrier oils we've talked about and what is on the market are decent sources of essential fatty acids, some oils are considered good sources of these vital nutrients.

Borage Oil – Taken from the seeds of a flowering perennial herb, borage oil is a potent source of omega-6 essential fatty acids. While we usually take omega-3 to counter the unhealthy balance of essential fatty acids that our diet affords, borage oil as a natural source is a different story.Omega-6, at its root, is actually as anti-inflammatory as omega-3, which likely aids in the topical benefits of borage oil. It's in the overconsumption of junk-food-sources and lack of balance in the omegas that we begin to see trouble.Borage oil has been used for dermatitis and other anti-inflammatory preparations.

Evening Primrose Oil – Named for the flowers that open only in the evenings, evening primrose oil is a more delicate oil that must be cold pressed, refrigerated, and should not be added to any heat preparations. Typically, evening primrose is consumed in supplement or culinary form, and of those uses it is highly researched and evaluated for its benefits as a source of essential fatty acids. For topical use, results seem to be similar to that of borage: anti-inflammatory effects that relieve flare ups such as dermatitis.

Although these are culinary oils, we already get large amounts of omega-6 in the diet. Be cautious with long-term culinary ingestion without professional guidance.

Choose these when: Resolving topical inflammation; essential fatty acid deficiency/imbalance is a problem. Creating hormone-balancing serums and women's health blends.

How to Use a Carrier Oil

For simple dilution purposes, start with small amounts of your carrier oil and work up as you become comfortable and have sanitary ways of storing your blend. Always place blends into heat-sanitized containers, particularly if they will stay there for any amount of time.

Start with 1 tsp of carrier oil, which roughly translates to 60-100 drops. Since it's oil we are dealing with, the assumption is that it will be closer to 60 than 100. You can assume 100 for extra safety and simple dilutions (1% = 1 drop), or you can calculate based on the more generous (and likely more accurate) 60.

A quick review from last chapter...

- 1% dilution = 6 drops of essential oils per 1 ounce of carrier oil = good for sensitive skin face, genitals, underarms, babies to toddlers
- 2-3% dilution = 12 – 18 drops of essential oil per 1 ounce of carrier oil = standard adult concentration for massage oils, creams and DIY recipes
- 5% – 10% dilution = 30 – 60 drops of essential oil per 1 ounce of carrier oil = more for acute conditions like infections. Don't use for more than a week at a time.

- 25% dilution = 150 drops of essential oils per 1 ounce of carrier = for one-time application like wart removal, scraps, cuts, and other wounds.
- 50% dilution = 1:1 ratio of carrier to essential oils = not recommended unless under the supervision of a trained professional.

Stir the essential oil into the carrier, then apply as indicated. And that's that! You've successfully diluted your essential oil and enjoyed the added benefit of a nourishing carrier oil.

Chapter 3
Ingesting Essential Oils: Are They Safe for Internal Use or Not

What do you think? Is ingesting essential oils safe? It should be no surprise that scientific research and traditional aromatherapy agree on their answers.

I'm not sure how it exactly happened, but somehow misguided people started to instill fear into essential oils users that these precious compounds are unsafe for internal use. I say "misguided" in the deepest respect, as I understand that we all have differing opinions, and I know that I'm going to get a lot of "love mail" for this chapter – hate mail sounds too ugly, doesn't it? :)

With that said, the more I learn about them, ingesting essential oils in therapeutic is not a common practice for me and my family. I still enjoy a drop of peppermint and cinnamon in my morning latte, or a drop of lemon in sparkling water with some liquid stevia as my special soda pop, but that's about it unless I'm battling some specific health condition. It has taken me a year of research & study and literally hundreds (if not thousands) of hours to get to this "revelation."

The key is dosage. One or two drops of lime essential oil in your guacamole that will be shared with 4 or 5 other people is not your concern. This is referred to as "culinary dose." The concern is when people are taking consuming 4, 5, or 6+ drops at a time. This is known as a "therapeutic dose." More on this below...

What Aromatherapists Really Say About Ingesting Essential Oils

I regularly get questions from people asking me about ingesting essential oils and I now understand why there's so much confusion. One myth breeds more myths. Innocent uncertainty breeds more uncertainty. And the vicious cycle continues.

The fact remains that there are no scientific, evidence-based, anatomical, physiological or logical reasons to say that all essentials oils are unsafe for human consumption. Paradoxically, aromatherapists are still at odds with each other on this point, which confuses the casual essential oil user all the more. With that said, rest assured that large professional organizations like *National Association for Holistic Aromatherapy (NAHA)* support safe, internal use.

In the words of NAHA, "Essential oils may be applied on the skin (dermal application), inhaled, diffused or taken internally. Each of these methods have safety issues which need to be considered." And this makes complete sense to me. Like anything we can easily overdo it, and we must remember a little goes a long way with regard to essential oils – especially internal use! We can also find several local and online schools that will certify you as an aromatherapist and learn how to practice safe, internal use.

The *Atlantic Institute of Aromatherapy* is one organization in particular that I have strongly aligned myself with as it is the oldest aromatherapy school continually run by a practicing aromatherapist. Their founder, Sylla Sheppard-Hanger, has over 40 years of client-based experience, and has been teaching classes in aromatherapy since 1985. The bottom line is that when an organization like this includes ingesting essential oils guidelines in their curriculum – with hundreds of case studies to support their recommendations – people should stop for a second a listen, don't you agree?

And let's not forget what the universally acclaimed text, *Essential Oil Safety: A Guide for Health Care Professionals*, repeatedly refers to "maximum oral dose" in relation to ingesting essential oils safely and effectively.

The thing that really throws me through a loop regarding people who speak out against ingesting essential oils is that they are in direct opposition of the dozens of human studies in the scientific literature and completely disregard the Food and Drug Administration. Yes, you read that correctly! According to the FDA, ingesting essential oils is safe for human consumption as flavor ingredients. For the exhaustive FDA-approved list of Generally Recognized As Safe (GRAS) oils see below.

Note: not all oils that are safe for ingestion are included in the FDA-approved GRAS list. I recommend that we use this list as a base point to start the conversation about what is and what is not safe because it all boils down to dosage.

Ingesting Essential Oils: Do's and Don'ts

Before I dive into some of the ways that ingesting essential oils can be done safely, there some "housekeeping" items we need to discuss. Here are some do's and don'ts.

DAILY DO'S:

1. Inhale essential oils in an essential oil diffuser, inhaler, spritzer and other fun ways.
2. Add essential oils in your daily body care regimen.
3. Be careful – and learn the basics.
4. Enjoy the good things in life! There's nothing like one drop of lemon or orange oil mixed with Solubol in a 32 ounce glass liter of sparkling water with some liquid stevia as a special soda pop treat.
5. Have fun & be empowered! Using essential oils and other natural therapies is a life-changing experience for most people and remember to enjoy the journey as you learn all about them!

DAILY DON'TS:

1. Ingesting essential oils for "prevention." This is wasteful and dangerous, and I was a victim of the take-a-drop-of-essential-oil under your tongue (or in your water) everyday myth until I irritated my esophagus and developed acid reflux! The more I learn about EOs, the less I consume them – only for specific health conditions, or my special soda. And, no, it doesn't matter how "pure" or "therapeutic" they are. Daily consumption is NOT the most effective (and medicinal) way to use them, and it has taken me 3 years of trial & error (lots of error) and literally hundreds (if not thousands) of research hours to get to this "revelation." So, please learn from my mistakes!

2. Think that each health condition within a specific body system should be approached the same way. Meaning this: even though peppermint is great for IBS and nausea, it should not be used for GERD. The *University of Maryland Medical Center* specifically warns that peppermint tea and essential oil can relax the esophageal sphincter and pose risks for those with reflux.

3. Believe that "there is an oil for that." Essential oils have changed my life so much that I have devoted much of my personal and professional lives to sharing the message that they are truly God's Medicine.

Seriously, I'm the "oil" guy and I've been blessed with the opportunity to be featured on countless health summits, conferences and documentaries. Yet, let's be real. Like anything, essential oils are limited by what they can and we should not fall into the trap that they are the end-all cure because misguided hope will disappoint.

Ok, now that we've cleaned house, let's get to work...

Tips for Ingesting Essential Oils

I have written about ingesting essential oils extensively in my book, The Healing Power of Essential Oils, and if you're looking for a thorough video on how to use them safely and effectively, you can check a free screening of my Essential Oils for Abundant Living Masterclass. In the meantime, suffice it to say that essential oils are extremely potent plant-based compounds and should be used with care.

Also known as "volatile organic compounds," essential oils are chemical compounds found in the bark, leaves, flowers, roots and rinds of plants, fruit, and trees. Interestingly, there are no vitamins or minerals in essential oils as they are made up of compounds that we learn about in organic chemistry class like terpene hydrocarbons (e.g. sesquiterpenes, which have been shown to cross the blood brain barrier) and oxygenated compounds (e.g aldehydes, ketones and esters, which all have unique effects on the human body).

The key to ingesting essential oils, and why we should consider them in our natural health regimens, is that they combat pathogens (harmful microorganisms), are a source of antioxidants (needed to prevent and cure disease), and have been shown to contain advanced healing properties in addition to cancer cell cytotoxicity amongst other things.

CULINARY DOSES (1-3 DROPS PER DISH)

The safest way to ingest essential oils is in culinary use. Cooking with essential oils is an extremely safe way to enjoy the health benefits as well as enhance the flavor of your food. Here are some ideas of how to get started.

- Use 1-2 drops of cilantro or coriander with 1-2 drops of lime, for example, goes wonderfully with your homemade guacamole.
- Try 1 drop of cumin in your curry next time. Or, 2 drops of black pepper in virtually anything savory!
- You could use cinnamon essential oil in a cake batter, for example, but you'd only need one drop for the whole batch vs. a tsp or more of the bark powder.
- Mix 1 drop in your morning latte. I particularly enjoy a drop of peppermint and cinnamon in my fat-burning matcha green tea latte.

Do remember, however, that oil and water do not mix, so simply adding a drop to your coffee will leave that drop undiluted. This is why you need to add an edible carrier oil like coconut oil first before and then mix into your latte!

THERAPEUTIC DOSES (UP TO 5-6 DROPS PER APPLICATION)

When ingesting essential oils is necessitated for therapeutic purposes, much more than a culinary dose needed. "Therapeutic" amounts require up to 5-6 drops of essential oil per dose. To do this safely, taking them in a gel capsule is the preferred method. Alternatively, you can add 3-4 drops of essential oil with one tablespoon of an edible carrier oil like olive or grapeseed or coconut oil and consume that way. This is what we do for our immune-boosting "flu" shots.

HOW TO MAKE GEL CAPSULES

The safest (and most effective) way to ingest essential oils for therapeutic purposes is to take them in capsules. Taken from my book, *The Healing Power of Essential Oils*, simply follow these instructions.

BASIC CAPSULE FORMULA
(Makes 1 dose)

INGREDIENTS
- 4 drops essential oils
- Organic, unrefined coconut oil or olive oil

SUPPLIES
- Pipette
- Size 00 vegetarian capsules

1. Using a pipette, drop the essential oils into the narrower bottom half of the capsule.
2. Use the pipette to fill the remaining space in the capsule with coconut or olive oil.
3. Fit the wider top half of the capsule over the bottom half and secure snugly.
4. Swallow a capsule immediately with water on an empty stomach. Take twice daily.
5. Use up to 2 weeks at a time.

* Note: Do not premake and store for future use.

FDA Approved GRAS Essential Oils

It is important to realize that millions of people are ingesting essential oils all day without even realizing it. Where do you think your processed food get their flavor from! Virtually anything that is naturally flavored most likely contains essential oils. This is what the FDA says in the official document Code of Regulations, Title 21, Volume 6, Animal Food Labeling: Specific Animal Food Labeling Requirements.

FOODS CONTAINING "ARTIFICIAL FLAVORS" AND "SPICES" DO NOT CONTAIN OILS

"The term artificial flavor or artificial flavoring means any substance, the function of which is to impart flavor, which is not derived from a spice, fruit or fruit juice, vegetable or vegetable juice, edible yeast, herb, bark, bud, root, leaf or similar plant material, meat, fish, poultry, eggs, dairy products, or fermentation products thereof. The term spice means any aromatic vegetable substance in the whole, broken, or ground form, except for those substances which have been traditionally regarded as foods, such as onions, garlic and celery; whose significant function in food is seasoning rather than nutritional; that is true to name; and from which no portion of any volatile oil or other flavoring principle has been removed.

- *Allspice, Anise, Basil, Bay leaves, Caraway seed, Cardamon, Celery seed, Chervil, Cinnamon, Cloves, Coriander, Cumin seed, Dill seed, Fennel seed, Fenugreek, Ginger, Horseradish, Mace, Marjoram, Mustard flour, Nutmeg, Oregano, Paprika, Parsley, Pepper, black; Pepper, white; Pepper, red; Rosemary, Saffron, Sage, Savory, Star aniseed, Tarragon, Thyme, Turmeric.*

- *Paprika, turmeric, and saffron or other spices which are also colors, shall be declared as spice and coloring unless declared by their common or usual name.*

FOODS CONTAINING "NATURAL FLAVORS" DO CONTAIN OILS

The term natural flavor or natural flavoring means the essential oil, oleoresin, essence or extractive, protein hydrolysate, distillate, or any product of roasting, heating or enzymolysis, which contains the flavoring constituents derived from a spice, fruit or fruit juice, vegetable or vegetable juice, edible yeast, herb, bark, bud, root, leaf or similar plant material, meat, seafood, poultry, eggs, dairy products, or fermentation products thereof, whose significant function in food is flavoring rather than nutritional. Natural flavors, include the natural essence or extractives obtained from plants." By letting common sense be our guide, I propose some tried and true tips on how to take essential oils internally.

1. Start off by using oils that are GRAS (see below for the FDA-approved list of oils that are Generally Recognized As Safe for internal use).
2. Be safe (more on that below).
3. Don't overdo it – limit to 2-3 drops at a time, and be sure to wait at least 4 hours before taking consecutive doses.
4. Listen to your body, and...
5. Discontinue use IMMEDIATELY if adverse reactions occur.

Trust me, people don't break out in hives in a "detox" reaction when ingesting essential oils like I've read out there in cyberspace. Pain, irritation, swelling, inflammation, bloating, burning, reflux, and anything else that isn't pleasant is NOT a good sign. This is your body's way of warning you that something harmful is attacking it.

[Code of Federal Regulations]
[Title 21, Volume 3]
[Revised as of April 1, 2015]
[CITE: 21CFR182.20]

TITLE 21–FOOD AND DRUGS

CHAPTER I–FOOD AND DRUG ADMINISTRATION DEPARTMENT OF HEALTH AND HUMAN SERVICES

SUBCHAPTER B–FOOD FOR HUMAN CONSUMPTION (CONTINUED)

PART 182 — SUBSTANCES GENERALLY RECOGNIZED AS SAFE Subpart A–General Provisions

Sec. 182.20 Essential oils, oleoresins (solvent-free), and natural extractives (including distillates).

Essential oils, oleoresins (solvent-free), and natural extractives (including distillates) that are generally recognized as safe for their intended use, within the meaning of section 409 of the Act, are as follows:

Common name	Botanical name of plant source
Alfalfa	Medicago sativa L.
Allspice	Pimenta officinalis Lindl.
Almond, bitter (free from prussic acid)	Prunus amygdalus Batsch, Prunus armeniaca L., or Prunus persica (L.) Batsch.
Ambrette (seed)	Hibiscus moschatus Moench.
Angelica root	Angelica archangelica L.
Angelica seed	Do.
Angelica stem	Do.
Angostura (cusparia bark)	Galipea officinalis Hancock.
Anise	Pimpinella anisum L.
Asafetida	Ferula assa-foetida L. and related spp. of Ferula.
Balm (lemon balm)	Melissa officinalis L.
Balsam of Peru	Myroxylon pereirae Klotzsch.
Basil	Ocimum basilicum L.
Bay leaves	Laurus nobilis L.
Bay (myrcia oil)	Pimenta racemosa (Mill.) J. W. Moore.
Bergamot (bergamot orange)	Citrus aurantium L. subsp. bergamia Wright et Arn.
Bitter almond (free from prussic acid)	Prunus amygdalus Batsch, Prunus armeniaca L., or Prunus persica (L.) Batsch.
Bois de rose	Aniba rosaeodora Ducke.
Cacao	Theobroma cacao L.
Camomile (chamomile) flowers, Hungarian	Matricaria chamomilla L.
Camomile (chamomile) flowers, Roman or English	Anthemis nobilis L.
Cananga	Cananga odorata Hook. f. and Thoms.
Capsicum	Capsicum frutescens L. and Capsicum annuum L.

Caraway	Carum carvi L.
Cardamom seed (cardamon)	Elettaria cardamomum Maton.
Carob bean	Ceratonia siliqua L.
Carrot	Daucus carota L.
Cascarilla bark	Croton eluteria Benn.
Cassia bark, Chinese	Cinnamomum cassia Blume.
Cassia bark, Padang or Batavia	Cinnamomum burmanni Blume.
Cassia bark, Saigon	Cinnamomum loureirii Nees.
Celery seed	Apium graveolens L.
Cherry, wild, bark	Prunus serotina Ehrh.
Chervil	Anthriscus cerefolium (L.) Hoffm.
Chicory	Cichorium intybus L.
Cinnamon bark, Ceylon	Cinnamomum zeylanicum Nees.
Cinnamon bark, Chinese	Cinnamomum cassia Blume.
Cinnamon bark, Saigon	Cinnamomum loureirii Nees.
Cinnamon leaf, Ceylon	Cinnamomum zeylanicum Nees.
Cinnamon leaf, Chinese	Cinnamomum cassia Blume.
Cinnamon leaf, Saigon	Cinnamomum loureirii Nees.
Citronella	Cymbopogon nardus Rendle.
Citrus peels	Citrus spp.
Clary (clary sage)	Salvia sclarea L.
Clover	Trifolium spp.
Coca (decocainized)	Erythroxylum coca Lam. and other spp. of Erythroxylum.
Coffee	Coffea spp.
Cola nut	Cola acuminata Schott and Endl., and other spp. of Cola.
Coriander	Coriandrum sativum L.
Cumin (cummin)	Cuminum cyminum L.
Curacao orange peel (orange, bitter peel)	Citrus aurantium L.
Cusparia bark	Galipea officinalis Hancock.

Dandelion	Taraxacum officinale Weber and T. laevigatum DC.
Dandelion root	Do.
Dog grass (quackgrass, triticum)	Agropyron repens (L.) Beauv.
Elder flowers	Sambucus canadensis L. and S. nigra l.
Estragole (estragole, esdragon, tarragon)	Artemisia dracunculus L.
Estragon (tarragon)	Do.
Fennel, sweet	Foeniculum vulgare Mill.
Fenugreek	Trigonella foenum-graecum L.
Galanga (galangal)	Alpinia officinarum Hance.
Geranium	Pelargonium spp.
Geranium, East Indian	Cymbopogon martini Stapf.
Geranium, rose	Pelargonium graveolens L'Her.
Ginger	Zingiber officinale Rosc.
Grapefruit	Citrus paradisi Macf.
Guava	Psidium spp.
Hickory bark	Carya spp.
Horehound (hoarhound)	Marrubium vulgare L.
Hops	Humulus lupulus L.
Horsemint	Monarda punctata L.
Hyssop	Hyssopus officinalis L.
Immortelle	Helichrysum angustifolium DC.
Jasmine	Jasminum officinale L. and other spp. of Jasminum.
Juniper (berries)	Juniperus communis L.
Kola nut	Cola acuminata Schott and Endl., and other spp. of Cola.
Laurel berries	Laurus nobilis L.
Laurel leaves	Laurus spp.
Lavender	Lavandula officinalis Chaix.
Lavender, spike	Lavandula latifolia Vill.

Lavandin	Hybrids between Lavandula officinalis Chaix and Lavandula latifolia Vill.
Lemon	Citrus limon (L.) Burm. f.
Lemon balm (see balm)	
Lemon grass	Cymbopogon citratus DC. and Cymbopogon lexuosus Stapf.
Lemon peel	Citrus limon (L.) Burm. f.
Lime	Citrus aurantifolia Swingle.
Linden flowers	Tilia spp.
Locust bean	Ceratonia siliqua L,
Lupulin	Humulus lupulus L.
Mace	Myristica fragrans Houtt.
Mandarin	Citrus reticulata Blanco.
Marjoram, sweet	Majorana hortensis Moench.
Mate	Ilex paraguariensis St. Hil.
Melissa (see balm)	
Menthol	Mentha spp.
Menthyl acetate	Do.
Molasses (extract)	Saccarum officinarum L.
Mustard	Brassica spp.
Naringin	Citrus paradisi Macf.
Neroli, bigarade	Citrus aurantium L.
Nutmeg	Myristica fragrans Houtt.
Onion	Allium cepa L.
Orange, bitter, flowers	Citrus aurantium L.
Orange, bitter, peel	Do.
Orange leaf	Citrus sinensis (L.) Osbeck.
Orange, sweet	Do.
Orange, sweet, flowers	Do.
Orange, sweet, peel	Do.
Origanum	Origanum spp.
Palmarosa	Cymbopogon martini Stapf.

Paprika	Capsicum annuum L.
Parsley	Petroselinum crispum (Mill.) Mansf.
Pepper, black	Piper nigrum L.
Pepper, white	Do.
Peppermint	Mentha piperita L.
Peruvian balsam	Myroxylon pereirae Klotzsch.
Petitgrain	Citrus aurantium L.
Petitgrain lemon	Citrus limon (L.) Burm. f.
Petitgrain mandarin or tangerine	Citrus reticulata Blanco.
Pimenta	Pimenta officinalis Lindl.
Pimenta leaf	Pimenta officinalis Lindl.
Pipsissewa leaves	Chimaphila umbellata Nutt.
Pomegranate	Punica granatum L.
Prickly ash bark	Xanthoxylum (or Zanthoxylum) Americanum Mill. or Xanthoxylum clava-herculis L.
Rose absolute	Rosa alba L., Rosa centifolia L., Rosa damascena Mill., Rosa gallica L., and vars. of these spp.
Rose (otto of roses, attar of roses)	Do.
Rose buds	Do.
Rose flowers	Do.
Rose fruit (hips)	Do.
Rose geranium	Pelargonium graveolens L'Her.
Rose leaves	Rosa spp.
Rosemary	Rosmarinus officinalis L.
Saffron	Crocus sativus L.
Sage	Salvia officinalis L.
Sage, Greek	Salvia triloba L.
Sage, Spanish	Salvia lavandulifolia Vahl.
St. John's bread	Ceratonia siliqua L.
Savory, summer	Satureia hortensis L.

Savory, winter	Satureia montana L.
Schinus molle	Schinus molle L.
Sloe berries (blackthorn berries)	Prunus spinosa L.
Spearmint	Mentha spicata L.
Spike lavender	Lavandula latifolia Vill.
Tamarind	Tamarindus indica L.
Tangerine	Citrus reticulata Blanco.
Tarragon	Artemisia dracunculus L.
Tea	Thea sinensis L.
Thyme	Thymus vulgaris L. and Thymus zygis var. gracilis Boiss.
Thyme, white	Do.
Thyme, wild or creeping	Thymus serpyllum L.
Triticum (see dog grass)	
Tuberose	Polianthes tuberosa L.
Turmeric	Curcuma longa L.
Vanilla	Vanilla planifolia Andr. or Vanilla tahitensis J. W. Moore.
Violet flowers	Viola odorata L.
Violet leaves	Do.
Violet leaves absolute	Do.
Wild cherry bark	Prunus serotina Ehrh.
Ylang-ylang	Cananga odorata Hook. f. and Thoms.
Zedoary bark	Curcuma zedoaria Rosc.

[42 FR 14640, Mar. 15, 1977, as amended at 44 FR 3963, Jan. 19, 1979; 47 FR 29953, July 9, 1982; 48 FR 51613, Nov. 10, 1983; 50 FR 21043 and 21044, May 22, 1985]

Chapter 4
Where to Buy Essential Oils and Choosing the Best Brand for You

Knowing where to buy essential oils isn't as simple as it may seem. Like choosing your doctor, you should be careful to not settle for anything but the best. I have done my best to help you navigate these often muddy waters, and I strongly recommend that you bookmark this page because it will serve to answer most of your questions about how to choose the best essential oils brands for your and your family!

By far, the #1 most common question I receive from the folks who get my weekly newsletter or follow me on Facebook is to which essential oil brand I recommend.

Interestingly, when choosing where to buy essential oils, fewer people ask for the brands that I recommend (emphasis on the pleural), which leads me to believe that most are trying to find the "Holy Grail" when they question me. In fact, snugged right next to this question, many people also ask me what the "best brand" is. Sadly, this train of thought has gotten a lot of people into trouble because nothing could be further from the truth.

Don't get me wrong, I really can't fault anyone for thinking this. We live in such a capitalist-driven society where we have been trained to believe that the competition is never as good as the "real deal." Not to mention, networking marketing companies have done an exceptionally thorough job reshaping the way that people view oils. The "brand wars" have reached fever pitch at this point, and people will swear on their deathbed that their brand sells the only pure oils on the market and all others are contaminated!

Again, I really can't fault people for thinking this. What else are they to logically think when a cancerous tumor disappears after using frankincense oil or their Lyme disease vanishes after using the protocol a distributor friend of theirs recommends?

Literally, there is no lack testimonials out there, and I personally know people who swear essential oils saved their lives. I'm not talking about bloggers out there who use their "story" to sell oils. No, I'm talking about real people with real testimonials about real essential oils! This is why it's so important to know where to buy essential oils.

What Every Blogger, Distributor & Mom Needs to Know and How to Buy Essential Oils

First off, as a public health researcher I am committed to staying as unbiased as possible so I don't give product recommendations when asked where to buy essential oils.

Not to mention, if I start selling and recommending essential oil brands, the Food and Drug Administration can shut down my website like they have several of my colleagues for making so-called "drug claims." Unlike pharmaceuticals, the manufacturing of EOs and supplements are not monitored by the government. This is why your medical doctor can recommend (and sell) specific drugs.

Things work differently in the natural health world. The only solace I have to continue educating the world about the life-transforming properties of natural therapies like essential oils is the First Amendment at this point. And, to maintain my freedom of speech to discuss what the scientific research has to say about how essential oils affect the body and various disease processes, I need to remain brand neutral about where to buy essential oils.

There are some good Facebook groups, however, that lay it all out there. The purpose of my work is not to dive into where to buy essential oils, but to educate about their uses. Once we start to name brands and recommend where to buy essential oils, we get into the FDA's scope and we want to preserve our freedom of speech. It's a fine line deciding where to buy essential oils.

With that said, let me break it to y'all. When considering where to buy essential oils, just realize that there is no #1 essential oils company. It simply does not, nor will it ever, exist.

Now, don't stone me because I refuse to bow down to the essential oil gods out there. If you've been following my work for a while, I hope that you've come to appreciate that my mission in life is not to give people fish, but to give them the fishing pole that they need to regain control of their health. As a Biblical health educator and public health researcher, I'm very passionate about educating people and equipping them to take the information that I teach about the next level of deciding where to buy essential oils.

The take home message about where to buy essential oils all boils down to trust. As you will see below, the entire supplement and essential oil industries are entirely built upon the "honor code." If you have found a company that you can put your faith in because they readily provide you with the information that you're looking for, your body responds well to their products, and you have no reason to believe that they are selling junk then you found a "keeper."

On the other hand, if you cannot get the information that you want from them a company, your body reacts to the oils in an undesirable manner and you develop suspicions because of an increase negative reports on the Internet, you should probably find a new brand that you can put your faith in.

With that said, let's now tackle the most emotionally-charged and controversial topic in the essential oils industry: where to buy essential oils!

6 Tips to Discovering the Right Brand for YOU

There are several quality, therapeutic grade brands out there and we use several of them. Here's what Mama Z and I do before we start using new essential oils:

1. Ask the company that you're investigating for a report of their sourcing and quality standards (check out the section "How to Check for Quality" below).
2. Contact a friend or family member who uses essential oils that you trust to be conscientious and a thorough researcher – be careful to not let hate speech and multi-level marketing propaganda get in the way of truth. EVERYONE's brand is the best, right? Especially, when they're selling something. ;)

3. Contact the company and see if they sell therapeutic grade oils, and ask them for a definition of what "therapeutic grade" means because this is an unregulated term that can be defined in a variety of ways.

4. Check to see if the oils are safe for internal use. Look for the SUPPLEMENT label on the bottle, which is an indication that the company you are interested in sells oils that are generally recognized as safe (GRAS). More on this below.

5. Try a couple, and test for yourself. Lemon, lavender and peppermint are common, relatively inexpensive and you should get a good gauge to see if this brand is for you or not.

6. Remember, many of the small companies get their oils from the same suppliers. They just private label them.

From what I've been told, the larger companies have unique suppliers, which differentiates their product from their competitor. This doesn't guarantee purity, but it can help put your mind to rest that they (should) be proprietary which should help you decide where to buy essential oils.

Note: For a product to be labeled as an "essential oil supplement," a supplemental fact label is required to be placed on the bottle, even though prior FDA approval is not required to use these labels. Essential oils that are being recommended for ingestion should have the supplemental fact labels on the bottle, however, this is not always the case. As well, the supplement label is not a guarantee of safety or purity as these labels are not regulated unless complaints or injury reports cause the FDA to intervene.

More on this below...

How to Buy Essential Oils: Quality Assessment

Before jumping in and buying a bunch of oils from a company, consider asking these questions to help ensure quality:

- Does the company has relations with their distillers?
- Can the company readily supply a batch-specific report (MS/GC) on the oil it sells?

- Can the company readily provide material safety data sheets (MSDS) upon request?
- What is the common name, latin name (exact genus and species), country of origin, part of plant processed, type of extraction (distillation or expression), and how it was grown (organic, wild-crafted, traditional)?

Also, it is critical to test for your own organoleptic assessment. "Organoleptic" meaning the way your body perceives the oil through the six senses: taste, touch, smell, vision, auditory, and intuition.

How to Buy Essential Oils: Indigenous Sourcing

In my opinion, the most important factor is whether or not the oils are indigenously sourced and organic in nature. Meaning, they are harvested where God planted them, which is why they are referred to as "native" plants. One reason why is because "organic" is not a guarantee of purity (more on that below). The other reason, and even more important, is because non-native plants pale in comparison to native plants when it come to nutrition and chemical constituency. This is something important to consider when deciding where to buy essential oils.

My father-in-law is a retired PhD agri scientist and spent his career evaluating the chemical compounds in plants. He told me that native plants always have a better nutritional profile because the soil is naturally designed to feed indigenous plants with what they need most. For example, we live in Atlanta, GA where the growing season lasts nearly 10 months out of the year. It's warm enough to sustain a fig tree in our backyard, but the taste and vitamin and mineral content of our fig is nothing what it should (and could) be if that same tree were grown in Israel where figs are native. Same for the pineapple, limes and lemons that grow in pots on our deck.

Additionally, there are some other importance differences between indigenous and non-indigenous plants when deciding where to buy essential oils:

NATIVE PLANTS

- Evolved over a long period of time, and best suited to thrive in their native region.
- Adapted to the local weather and geology.
- Can thrive in drought and inclement weather situations.
- Environmentally sustainable for pesticide-free farming because they have developed natural resistance to native predators.
- Has a positive impact on the local environment and ecosystem by forming natural "communities" with other plants.

NON-NATIVE PLANTS

- Unnaturally introduced (deliberately or by accident) into an environment in which they did not evolve.
- Are not well-suited for pesticide-free farming because they are not naturally resistant to native predators.
- Has a negative impact on the local environment and ecosystem because they have a tendency to take over a habitat, require pesticides to thrive, and are not natural food sources for neighboring wildlife.

Bottom line: organic in nature and indigenously sourced are best. This is important to remember when deciding where to buy essential oils.

How to Buy Essential Oils: Contamination Concerns

The fact that people are questioning which brands are best is a good thing. When considering where to buy essential oils, underlying concern and motivating factor is that people want to use unadulterated pure oils, with no contaminants or harmful fillers. I validate this concern 100% and hope that more people will demand pure products in the supplement world so that suppliers step up their game.

Remember, it's all about supply-and-demand.

Is Certified Organic Necessary?

In 2014, scientists and essential oil producers met at the International Federation of Essential Oil and Aroma Trades (IF EAT) Conference in Rome, Italy to share their concerns about quality and safety of our global essential oil supply. These are some of the key takeaways as shared by the Founder, President, CEO, and Principal of the American College of Healthcare Sciences (ACHS) Dorene Petersen:

- "Pesticide residue and concern for pesticide levels in essential oils, even in certified organic oils, was the subject of three sessions at IFEAT 2014."
- "It is a regrettable fact that essential oils can contain pesticide residues, even certified organic essential oils."
- "Detecting residue is even more likely if pesticides are administered during cultivation of the plant material."
- "However, passive contamination can also occur even if a farmer does not actively use pesticides."
- "Acts of nature such as a puff of wind or water runoff from a neighboring field, even incorrect storage of an essential oil, can all result in cross contamination."
- "According to the test results conducted by the German Medicines Manufacturers' Association (BAH) Working Group on Contaminants, cold-pressed essential oils from the pericarp of citrus fruits are more likely to contain pesticide residues than steam-distilled citrus because of the hydrophilic, thermostable, and volatile characteristics of pesticides."
- "Most pesticides can easily combine with or dissolve in lipids or fats, facilitating the transition to the oil."

The reality is that it's increasingly becoming more difficult to find truly pure, clean air, food and water because of modern agricultural methods and pollution on a global, massive scale. This is especially true for supplements and essential oils that are labelled "organic."

According to Petersen's report of the IFEAT meeting, it's all not doom-and-gloom.

The European Pharmacopoeia expert group database focused on essential oils from 2006 to 2013, have tested nearly 600 samples for 217 substances representing 28 different oils.

- 314 samples didn't show any residues.
- 275 samples were contaminated with at least one residue.
- 1,150 results were discovered to contain at least one pesticide residue.
- A few of the specific oils they looked at were neroli, rosemary, eucalyptus, caraway, and lavender.
- Of the 65 samples of neroli, 199 positive pesticide findings were discovered, and 77 showed that the pesticides were above the maximum levels.
- 49 samples of rosemary were tested, and 15 revealed more than the maximum level of a citrus peel treatment agent known as biphenyl.
- Interesting, rosemary does not have a peel so the presence of biphenyl can only be explained because it was contaminated by the packaging, the manufacturing equipment or some other man-made intervention.
- 36 eucalyptus and 25 caraway samples were tested, and three of each were positive for pesticides.
- 19 lavender samples tested and one was positive.

Bottom line: certified organic in good, but no guarantee for purity. Organic in nature is probably your best bet.

Essential Oil Regulation

At this point, the most natural question you should be asking is, "Who regulates essential oils?"

The easiest answer to this question is, "No one."

Technically-speaking, they are regulated in a roundabout way, but manufacturers and distributors are not required to obtain FDA approval to sell their products beforehand, so what's the purpose? "Because dietary supplements are under the "umbrella" of foods, FDA's Center for Food Safety and Applied Nutrition (CFSAN) is responsible for the agency's oversight of these products. DSHEA created a new regulatory framework for the safety and labeling of dietary supplements. FDA is not authorized to review dietary supplement products for safety and effectiveness before they are marketed."

Hence, the reason why you'll see this disclaimer on essential oil bottles, "*These statements have not been evaluated by the Food and Drug Administration. This product is not intended to diagnose, treat, cure, or prevent disease."

Unlike drugs, supplements and essential oils are not intended to cure, diagnose, prevent, or treat diseases. That means supplements should not make claims, such as "reduces pain" or "treats heart disease." Statements like these (i.e. "drug claims") can only be made for drugs, not essential oils or supplements.

Under the FD&C Act, cosmetic products and ingredients, with the exception of color additives, do not require FDA approval before they go on the market. Drugs, however, must generally either receive premarket approval by the FDA through the New Drug Application (NDA) process or conform to a "monograph" for a particular drug category, as established by FDA's Over-the-Counter (OTC) Drug Review. These monographs specify conditions whereby OTC drug ingredients are generally recognized as safe and effective, and not misbranded. Certain OTC drugs may remain on the market without an NDA approval until a monograph for its class of drugs is finalized as a regulation.

When choosing where to buy essential oils, it's important to keep in mind that they are only regulated after they go to market. Even then, in the tangled web of "regulation" there are so many loopholes that there is virtually no system set in place to properly regulate the products being sold. To help make sense of this all, here is a quick summary of the current regulatory system and the principal players:

1. The Dietary Supplement Health and Education Act (DSHEA) of 1994, which amended the Federal Food, Drug, and Cosmetic Act, regulates manufacturers by holding them accountable to what are known as "good manufacturing practices" (i.e., industry qual-

ity standards).

2. The Food and Drug Administration (FDA) regulates the label, but only after the product goes to market. (More on this below...).

3. The Federal Trade Commission (FTC) regulates supplement advertising – manufacturers must report truthfully what their products contain and must have proof backing up any claims they make.

4. Dietary Supplement and Nonprescription Drug Consumer Protection Act (DSNDCPA) of 2006 requires "adverse event reporting" – the same system the FDA uses to inform the public about injury reports and unsafe incidents.

Under the DSHEA, the FDA is responsible for uncovering what supplements are "unsafe" before it can remove the products from the marketplace. Essentially, all essential oils and supplements are innocent until proven guilty and the primary way the FDA is aware of a situation necessitating an investigation is at the very hands of the manufacturers and distributors themselves; as they are required to record, investigate and forward all safety concerns and adverse event reports to the FDA.

Drug Claims

In contrast to dietary supplement manufacturers, who are able to utilize structure/function claims, aromatherapy companies who sell essential oils for external use cannot.

Establishing a Product's Intended Use

"A product can be a drug, a cosmetic, or a combination of both... For example, a fragrance marketed for promoting attractiveness is a cosmetic. But a fragrance marketed with certain 'aromatherapy' claims, such as assertions that the scent will help the consumer sleep or quit smoking, meets the definition of a drug because of its intended use. Similarly, a massage oil that is simply intended to lubricate the skin and impart fragrance is a cosmetic, but if the product is intended for a therapeutic use, such as relieving muscle pain, it's a drug."

This is where some brands get in trouble because they, or their distributors, make "drug claims" that are outside the scope of cosmetics. "The law doesn't require cosmetics to have FDA approval before they go on the market. But FDA can take action against a cosmetic on the market if we have reliable information showing that it is unsafe when consumers use it according to directions on the label, or in the customary or expected way, or if it is not labeled properly."

THE SUPPLEMENT LABEL AND INTERNAL USE

Essentially, if the label says SUPPLEMENT, then yes, it's considered a consumable product. This is something to keep in minding when considering where to buy essential oils.

As described by the U.S. Food and Drug Administration, "A dietary supplement is a product intended for ingestion that contains a 'dietary ingredient' intended to add further nutritional value to (supplement) the diet. A 'dietary ingredient' may be one, or any combination, of the following substances:

- a vitamin
- a mineral
- an herb or other botanical
- an amino acid
- a dietary substance for use by people to supplement the diet by increasing the total dietary intake
- a concentrate, metabolite, constituent, or extract

Dietary supplements may be found in many forms such as tablets, capsules, softgels, gelcaps, liquids, or powders. Some dietary supplements can help ensure that you get an adequate dietary intake of essential nutrients; others may help you reduce your risk of disease."

Other sources like *Jade Shutes from the School for Aromatic Studies* explain this further: *"Dietary supplements can be created by using both nutritive and non-nutritive ingredients. Essential oils, of course, would be considered non-nutritive dietary supplements. The use of essential oils continues to actually grow within the dietary supplement world. This is the value of GRAS approved essential oils. They have already gone through incredible safety evaluation for internal use. So we see dietary supplement companies utilizing GRAS approved essential oils/co2 extracts."*

Remember that essential oils are oftentimes a key component of the supplements that we take, and this is key: Dietary supplement manufacturers are able to utilize structure/function claims whereas traditional aromatherapy companies who sell essential oils for external application cannot.

So, if a company states on the bottle or package that their essential oil product(s) can alter body function (i.e. reduce pain, inflammation, etc.), the FDA requires that these claims be supported by conclusive evidence to prove the supplement truly has the claimed effect. These types of claims on labels must be approved by the FDA within 30 days after its first use. Additionally, the FDA requires that this information be printed on the product label in a clear manner for it to be regulated. Still then, these claims can only be "general structure function" and cannot state the product "cures" or "treats" a disease or illness.

This seems pretty straightforward, but is not a guarantee that products are being regulated. Only products that make claims on them are regulated. So, the natural course of action for a vast majority of supplement and essential oils' manufacturers is to simply not make claims on their labels! Then, these same companies can make claims on their website and try to walk this fine line and stay under the FDA's radar. For instance, let's say that:

- Company XYZ states that a product reduces pain and inflammation on their website only.
- Company XYZ does NOT state this on their dietary fact supplement label.
- Subsequently, the label does NOT require FDA approval before it goes to market.
- The supplement label will be regulated by the FDA ONLY if it has been found to be adulterated or responsible of causing harm.
- If dietary supplement claims are made on a supplement label, Company XYZ is then required to have substantiating evidence to back up their claim and get approval within 30 days after its first use.

The bottom line is that according to the law (DSHEA), manufacturers are responsible for ensuring that their products are safe before they are marketed; which is a main factor when considering where to buy essential oils.

Watch a FREE Screening of My 10-Part Video Masterclass to Transform Your Home (and Life!) with Essential Oils... Reserve Your Spot Today!

EssentialOilsForAbundantLiving.com

Looking for More?

Join Dr. Z's Essential Oils Club for Monthly Q & A's, Expert Interviews & More!

EssentialOilsClub.info

Other Books By Dr. Z:

The Healing Power of Essential Oils
HealingPowerOfEssentialOils.com

The Essential Oils Diet
EssentialOilsDiet.com

Section 2
Essential Oils and Gut Health

Chapter 5
Maximizing Gut Health with Essential Oils

We've been hard on our digestive system for decades, and it's only getting worse. Not only does the food (and drink) we consume play a direct role, but lifestyle factors right down to how stressed we feel can dole out damage to the gut. We know that using essential oils for stomach health can be beneficial, but what if the damage is already done? If you are an adult in our society, chances are, how to heal your gut naturally applies to you!

As some of the most intriguing and powerful components of herbal material, essential oils can be used as a tool for gut health to help heal the damaged gut...

How to Heal Your Gut Naturally with Essential Oils: 5 Gut Health Problems

Sometimes, an individual's gut can be damaged without their knowledge. Perhaps the bacterial balance is off and the immune system is faltering. Maybe their emotions swing wildly, or cognitive function falters, and knowing how to heal your gut naturally is vital information.

The gut is a command post for much of the body, with nervous system transmitters that rival the CNS in the brain and spinal cord. So even if you don't think you have gut health problems – or you think you have unrelated issues – it's worth looking at your history, lifestyle, and dietary choices to consider whether you have damaged your gut in any way.

For everyone else, you know you have gut health troubles and you need to know how to heal your gut naturally, because it manifests in uncomfortable, or often painful ways.

Essential oils for gut health aren't always the perfect match for every gut health imbalance, but there are definite cases where their use is indicated and even preferred.

1) LEAKY GUT

Leaky Gut Syndrome is a common gastrointestinal problem that has been gathering a lot of attention lately because research continues to link it to a number of other health issues and diseases. The SAD (Standard American Diet), stress, toxic overload and bacterial imbalance people battle has certainly contributed to the epidemic that now affects millions of people globally, and if you're one of them, you want to know how to heal your gut naturally.

The gut is tricky to treat because it's so far down the GI tract so leaky gut is a good one to start off with. The only way to ensure that essential oils can reach the gut is to use an enteric-coated capsule.

- Peppermint and caraway have been proven to soothe information like no other blend – taken internally. This combination is also highly effective at promoting healthy gastrointestinal motility.
- Thymol and carvacrol (thyme and oregano) are fantastic for promoting intestinal integrity and immune responses.
- Additionally, oregano essential oil has been proven to repair the gut lining– thus preventing chemicals from leaking out of the gut.

All these can be applied topically over the abdomen. 2-3x per day. At a 2-5% dilution depending on the oils used and their recommended max dermal limits.

2) SIBO & DYSBIOSIS

The microbial balance in the gut can be shifted in many ways, usually categorized as dysbiosis. A particularly concerning form of dysbiosis is that of SIBO (Small Intestine Bacterial Overgrowth), which occurs when bacteria that should be in the colon are found in the small intestine. Both generalized dysbiosis and the more specific condition of SIBO are connected with other health concerns, including IBS and metabolic disorders.

Essential oils for stomach health are indicated for SIBO and other gut flora issues when the essential oil is able to exhibit symptom relief without damaging beneficial bacteria. In 2012, a study analyzing the development of a probiotic (beneficial bacteria in supplement form) found certain essential oils to work well with the formula, creating a synergistic effect of increased benefits.

A few years before that, eight essential oils for stomach health were analyzed for their effects on gut dysbiosis (bacterial imbalance). The findings included caraway, lavender, and neroli as stand-out examples of essential oils that would harmonize well with the beneficial bacteria in the body. These studies demonstrate the excellent ability that these essential oils have to affect detrimental bacteria while remaining gentle on the body and beneficial strains. Further research for dosing and ideal treatment methods of how to heal your gut naturally will be exciting to see!

Consuming enteric-coated peppermint capsules (3-6 drops per dose with an edible carrier oil) has also been shown to soothe inflammation and help SIBO patients considerably.

3) IBS

Irritable Bowel Syndrome was once considered little more than a non-diagnosis – the blanket term given when doctors essentially had no idea what was going on. Now, we know that IBS not only affects more than 10% of the global population, but that fewer than 30% of those affected will ever make it to the doctor to even seek a diagnosis. IBS is usually managed with diet and medication, but essential oils – especially in enteric coated capsules that can make it past the stomach – have been indicated for symptom control, as well.

Although more extensive studies are welcomed, an extensive review conducted in 2008 shows peppermint oil exhibiting significant improvement over placebo, alongside dietary fiber – both of which stood alongside antispasmodic medications in efficacy. To ensure the oil reaches the intestines, enteric coated capsule preparations are indicated by studies.

4) GERD

While the "gut" is technically the intestines, we usually use it interchangeably with the digestive system as a whole. As such, health trouble can start as quickly as the esophagus and acid reflux or GERD. This combination problem is related to stomach acids (both too much and too little) as well as a faulty "flap" that should keep the acid out of the esophagus. Acid levels can be affected by lifestyle and diet, as well as bacteria. One way to approach GERD with essential oils for stomach health is to use oils that protect the stomach and improve digestive processes.

Ginger fits the bill, in tandem with turmeric, as indicated in a study released in January 2015. The researchers tested antioxidant levels in rats with and without turmeric and ginger essential oils. The oils seemed to increase antioxidant levels as well as reduce damage done to the stomach wall. Culinary preparations would make sense here, providing a digestive system boost to your regular mealtime.

Applying a 5% dilution of ginger over your abdomen and chest can help with acid reflux!

5) NAUSEA

Within the stomach, nausea is another common problem, associated with a number of ailments as a symptom ranging from unpleasant to debilitating. Anyone who has experience nausea knows that scent has a major effect on how you feel, in either a positive or negative manner. Inhaled essential oils for stomach health are an excellent tool for managing nausea of nearly any cause.

Backing this up with promising research, we see that peppermint and ginger work well together for alleviating nausea. Refreshing citrus oils can also be beneficial, with lemon standing out as helpful for dreaded morning sickness nausea in pregnancy.

Carrying around personal inhalers with a mixture of lemon, peppermint and ginger may be trick to help in moments of queasiness.

Healing the Gut

We can't discuss gut health or healing remedies without discussing the importance of bacteria. Totaling more of our body composition by weight than our own cells, bacteria comprise a formidable ally or opponent, depending on the situation.

In a journal article describing the importance of gut flora, researchers detailed the "collective metabolic activity equal to a virtual organ within an organ," created by bacterial populations in the body.

If you're squirming in your seat at all of this talk of bacteria, you've probably internalized the "kills 99.9% of bacteria" line that keeps us from caring about our microscopic partners in health. More likely than not, you also have gut damage to heal.

Without restoring or protecting the bacterial balance in the gut, remedies and healing techniques will be ineffective or short lived or both. Fortunately, digestive-wellness essential oils are typically safe, and will presumably be used as part of an overall shift toward holistic wellness.

Be sure you don't discount the importance of gut health because it is responsible for a vast majority of your immune function! From a seminal 2008 report:

> *The gastrointestinal system plays a central role in immune system homeostasis. It is the main route of contact with the external environment and is overloaded every day with external stimuli, sometimes dangerous as pathogens (bacteria, protozoa, fungi, viruses) or toxic substances, in other cases very useful as food or commensal flora.*
>
> **The crucial position of the gastrointestinal system is testified by the huge amount of immune cells that reside within it.** Indeed, gut-associated lymphoid tissue (GALT) is the prominent part of mucosal-associated lymphoid tissue (MALT) and **represents almost 70% of the entire immune system; moreover, about 80% of plasma cells [mainly immunoglobulin A (IgA)-bearing cells] reside in GALT.**

GALT interacts strictly with gastrointestinal functions in a dynamic manner; for instance, by increasing intestinal permeability in reply to particular stimulations, or orientating the immune response towards luminal content, allowing either tolerance or elimination/ degradation of luminal antigens, or sometimes provoking damage to the intestinal mucosa, such as in coeliac disease or food allergy.

Promoting Gut Health with Essential Oils

While these oils carry evidence of benefit to overall gut health and can facilitate gut healing, do use caution when approaching disease states. As we all know, natural products are "not intended to diagnose, treat, cure, or prevent any disease."

Essential oils for stomach health are powerful and should be treated with the respect they deserve. If you have or suspect a disease or chronic ailment, seek a doctor and professional for advice.

With that out of the way, let's highlight some of the gut healing benefits of essential oils, as backed by science.

- **Peppermint** – Like its parent plant, peppermint essential oil is known for its digestive remedy capabilities. Peppermint has long been indicated for IBS via enteric-coated capsules. This was revisited in 2013, with coriander and lemon balm mentioned for their effectiveness, as well.
- **Ginger** - Like peppermint, ginger essential oil can be your gut health VIP. It's very safe to consume (gel capsule, enteric-coated capsule) and works wonders topically.
- **Thyme** – An antimicrobial by day, gut healer by night, thyme is a superhero in the world of gut health. For SIBO, thymol and geraniol have been shown "effective in suppressing pathogens in the small intestine, with no concern for beneficial commensal colonic bacteria in the distal gut." Thymol, of course, is the major component of thyme, while geraniol is found in high concentrations in rose oil.
- **Lavender** – Not only have we seen lavender as effective against dysbiosis, but it is a well-reputed source of anti-inflammatory and healing properties. Additionally – perhaps not coincidentally –

lavender has been one of the most effective anxiolytic (anti-anxiety) essential oils, tested as a commercial internal preparation. Whether the anxiety was calmed due to improved gut health or it's just a convenient double purpose, lavender is a key component of nearly any healing protocol.

- **Cumin** – A recent study on IBS symptoms and essential oil treatments evaluated a 2% preparation of cumin essential oil in 57 patients with IBS. At the end of the four week maximum trial, symptoms including pain, bloating, and elimination problems were significantly decreased. Note – the level of cumin in the study was higher than the recommended dermal max (recommended 0.4%), however we can see the benefits this oil can offer.

This, of course, is just a highlight of the digestive oils. Ginger stands out for nausea and initial digestive complaints. Citrus oils are gentle and effective for both digestion and peripheral issues, like anxiety and microbial concerns. If you're serious about rebuilding your gut, essential oils should be near the top of your toolbox, researched and ready to go.

More Essential Oils for Gut Health

With a shift in focus away from eliminating dangerous bacteria and toward strengthening good bacteria, holistic options are available to us.

Holistic refers to the body as a whole, which means we can take those first baby steps toward wellness from any area of our lives. Diet is a primary concern, improving the gut directly via the substances that come in contact with it – particularly in light of many meat sources relying on gross misuse of antibiotics that may be retained in the meat itself. Cleaning supplies that do not harshly eliminate beneficial bacteria are also important, as well.

Believe it or not, even stress plays a role in gut health. A Harvard educational article describes this phenomenon as the "brain-gut axis," explaining,

> *The enteric nervous system is sometimes referred to as a "second brain" because it relies on the same types of neurons and neurotransmitters that are found in the central nervous system (brain*

and spinal cord)... researchers are interested in understanding how psychological or social stress might cause digestive problems.

Essential oils, if you haven't heard, can meet each of these needs – from improving the intestinal tract directly to cleaning up our cleaning products to relieving stress. If you're ready to be good to your gut, get these oils:

- Thyme & Rose
- Cardamom
- Clove
- Tea Tree & Oregano
- Fennel
- Tarragon

Each of their preparations and actions are different, but the overarching effects spell wellness for the gut. Here are some of the best ways to use these essential oils for gut health.

More Essential Oils for Gut Health

- **Thyme & Rose** – In a study released earlier this year, researchers found that the primary constituents of thyme and rose oil – thymol and geraniol, respectively – "could be effective in suppressing pathogens in the small intestine, with no concern for beneficial commensal colonic bacteria in the distal gut."

- **Cardamom** – Both anti-inflammatory and antispasmodic, cardamom is a soothing oil related to the ginger family. It has been associated with many digestive health benefits, including gastro-protective effects.

- **Clove** – As an oil with some of the most eugenol, clove is an efficient antimicrobial that can counter Candida albicans overgrowth. Its effects against the yeast are effective to the point that an over the counter internal preparation is being studied using clove oil.

- **Tea Tree & Oregano** – A powerful duo, tea tree and oregano essential oils are the case-in-point for antibacterial as a beneficial component, compared against harsher, synthetic or toxic antibacterials. Use in DIY cleaners to help stop the spread of viral illnesses without attempting to bleach away the good with the bad.

- **Fennel** – Used as a digestive stimulant in whole-herb form, the essential oil retains some of the soothing components for the gut as an antispasmodic, likely connected to the estragole content. This component is also found in fennel. Aromatherapy and diluted topical use are very popular, but since estragole has been monitored for potential toxicity internally some recommend against ingesting it.

- **Tarragon**: And, don't forget about tarragon. It's a super healing oil that promotes gut health as well!

Chapter 6
DIY Essential Oil Protocol for Gut Health

Now that we've talked about essential oils for gut health and oils that can help to heal the gut, we can walk through ways to use DIY essential oil blends for digestive issues. There are dozens of oils and countless blends out there, but a few are especially beneficial for the gut, with several approaches for application and use.

Most essential oils are helpful for fast-acting results, such as symptom relief and antimicrobial effects. This kind of effect matches well with gut health concerns and is amplified as part of a multipronged approach to healing the gut. Diet and lifestyle changes are imperative, and it's often worth working with a holistic healthcare professional to maximize your natural efforts using essential oils.

Taking a Whole-Body Approach Using a DIY Essential Oil Blend

As we walk through some of the uses for essential oils and gut health, it's important to remember that you can integrate the essential oils into your whole-body approach to wellness. Suggesting a DIY essential oil protocol or preparation does not exclude other steps toward health and healing.

For gut health in particular, a DIY essential oil blend will pair very well with probiotics, an absolutely vital component of intestinal healing and balance. They are also often used alongside digestive enzymes to maximize digestion improvement. An excellent example of early research on the combination comes with lab testing, where animals showed decreased intestinal inflammation with thymol and cinnamaldehyde essential oil components combined with the enzymes xylanase and beta-glucanase.

DIY Essential Oil Applications for the Gut

EOs can be used in numerous ways, varying based on the oil, individual, concern, and even preference. Here are some ways to use essential oils for improved gut health.

INTERNAL USE OF A DIY ESSENTIAL OIL

Use capsules when you need the oil to make it to the stomach rather than the mucous membranes of the esophagus. If the oil is specifically for the intestines, enteric coated capsules are necessary, which you can find, but they can be pricey.

The important thing to remember for capsule creation is that the oils should still be diluted as an extra precaution and to increase bioavailability (your body's ability to absorb plant-based compounds), and that the capsule shouldn't be filled only with the DIY essential oil blend for gut health. You still only need 2-3 drops at a time, so most of the capsule should be comprised of the carrier oil. Very small capsules (Size 00) are best.

Note: Internal, medicinal use of oils should be executed in proper dosing, with knowledge of contraindications and safe usage. Seek guidance or further education before creating and using capsules, or use a pre-formulated, pre-dosed essential oil supplement.

- *Optimal oils for capsule use*: peppermint, clove, ginger, oregano, tea tree, thyme. (Choose 2-3 oils at a time, and mix up protocol every couple weeks).

- *Optimal situations for capsule use*: indigestion, nausea, SIBO, leaky gut, IBS, GERD, dysbiosis, with supervision by an integrative care professional. (Note: **Peppermint oil could make GERD worse** and is not recommended for this specific condition.)

- *Carrier oil options*: coconut, almond, sesame, apricot kernel, avocado, castor, evening primrose, jojoba, sunflower, pumpkin seed, neem, hemp seed, hazelnut, borage seed.

TOPICAL USES OF A DIY ESSENTIAL OIL

The soothing effects of aromatherapy are translated well into massages, and an upset tummy can be eased with a topical application. If you keep a diluted blend or two on hand, you can quickly grab it and apply when needed.

Dilute oils to 1-3% of the total volume into a carrier oil of your choice. Favorites include coconut oil, almond oil, jojoba, and avocado oil. Do remember that if the coconut oil is exposed to temperatures below the mid-seventies, it will solidify. Fractionated coconut oil is an option if you'd like it to remain liquid and other carriers are unavailable.

- **Optimal oils for topical use:** peppermint, ginger, caraway, coriander, *fennel, anise, tarragon, thyme, or citrus.
- **Optimal situations for topical use**: indigestion, constipation, stomach aches, and nausea.
- **Word of Caution**: *Fennel oil (Foeniculum vulgare) contains the estrogenic compound Trans Anethole. This raises obvious concerns for people with estrogen dominance and estrogen positive cancer. Also, "estragole, a main component of vulgare has become a cause of concern, as the structurally similar methyleugenol has been recently found to be a potential carcinogen. This has led to the European Union (EU) to allow a new legal limit for estragole of 10 mg/kg in non-alcoholic beverages."

INHALATION

Don't let a pretty scent fool you! Aromatherapy is powerful, transferring the oil's composition to your body simply by inhaling it. Inhalation is actually one of, if not the most, effective ways to administer the benefits of essential oils.

We are most familiar with diffusion, but DIY essential oils for digestive health can be inhaled much more directly for the person who is experiencing tummy trouble or gut concerns. A couple of drops in a bowl of hot water becomes an instant personal steamer if you "tent" a towel over and inhale. Jewelry or clothing can hold a drop or two for a more lasting personal source to inhale, and aroma sticks can fit in pockets or purses for easy, portable access. The easiest method? Simply open the bottle and sniff!

- **Optimal oils for inhalation**: citrus, ginger, fennel, peppermint, clove, cinnamon...or any!
- **Optimal situations for inhalation**: nausea, stomach ache.

Note: It is recommended to avoid hot oils like cinnamon and clove in steam inhalations so as not to irritate the sinus passages.

DIY Essential Oil Digestive Blends

Now that you have a good idea of your options, you can start to connect them for overall health and wellness. Blending the oils first into a carrier oil or honey will ensure proper dispersion and dilution, creating a safer and more effective remedy. For internal use, culinary or otherwise, a pure, organic essential oil is ideal.

HEALTHY DIGESTION BLEND

- Choose a few of the following, and blend a total of 20 drops into 10 ml honey and carrier oil (coconut is my favorite): clove, orange, cinnamon, rosemary, eucalyptus, lemon. Stir 2 drops of this diluted blend into tea or water, or take directly.
- Add a drop or two of the following organic essential oils as replacements in culinary preparations: ginger, fennel, dill, coriander, cardamom, cinnamon, citrus, thyme, clove, etc.

NAUSEA BLEND

- Blend 3 drops ginger and 2 drops lemon and diffuse. You could also blend the same number of drops into 10ml carrier oil and apply topically.
- Blend 3 drops peppermint and 2 drops ginger and diffuse. You could also blend the same number of drops into 10ml carrier oil and apply topically.

TUMMY TROUBLE BLEND

- Choose a few of the following, and blend a total of 5 drops into 10ml carrier oil: cardamom, peppermint, tea tree, ginger, caraway, coriander, or fennel. Inhale or use topically.
- Blend one drop of peppermint and ginger in 1 tsp of honey and consume for soothed and improved digestion, or create capsules replacing the honey with carrier oil.

To recap from the chapters above:

- Oregano capsules can help repair Leaky Gut.
- Peppermint capsules can help soothe SIBO & IBS.
- Ginger is the all-around MVP. Topical and internal (capsules) work wonders for general nauseas, gas and bloating.

A working knowledge of DIY essential oil blends can be a valuable ally in times of digestive upset. Take the time to learn about each of these oils thoroughly so that you can add them to your at-home DIY essential oil medicine cabinet and begin to heal your gut.

Watch a FREE Screening of My 10-Part Video Masterclass to Transform Your Home (and Life!) with Essential Oils... Reserve Your Spot Today!

EssentialOilsForAbundantLiving.com

Looking for More?

Join Dr. Z's Essential Oils Club for Monthly Q & A's, Expert Interviews & More!

EssentialOilsClub.info

Other Books By Dr. Z:

The Healing Power of Essential Oils
HealingPowerOfEssentialOils.com

The Essential Oils Diet
EssentialOilsDiet.com

Section 3

Gut Healing Essential Oil Profiles

Chapter 7
5 Health Benefits of Anise Oil

With its licorice-reminiscent flavor and scent, anise brings a refreshing and unique element to your single-oil use or combination blends. Here, we'll learn how to differentiate true anise oil uses and incorporate them into your wellness routines.

Anise Plant Profile

When a common name is shared between plants, we often make the mistake of assuming they are related, similar, or even interchangeable. None of the above are necessarily true. Anise and star anise are examples, sharing the common name of anise, but they are entirely different plants. Latin names help us to narrow down exactly which plants we are dealing with and understand how to use them.

True anise is the plant of focus today, with the Latin name *Pimpinella anisum*. It's part of the dill family, a group of almost spindly annual and sometimes perennial herbs with "umbel" shaped flowering heads and strong aromatic compounds.

Star anise, on the other hand, is *Ilicium verum*, a spice derived from the pods of an evergreen tea.

Whole Herb Use

Anise seeds are usually the part of the plant used, and have been for generations. Traditional medicine uses anise seeds for *"carminative, aromatic, disinfectant, and galactagogue"* purposes, as well as menstrual issues, diabetes, inflammation, and more digestive issues.

A good example of anise whole-herb use is found in a 2007 article in the *World Journal of Gastroenterology*. An extract of the seeds was prepared and tested on gastrointestinal health. The researchers found that it could protect the gut against ulcers and lesions, perhaps thanks to its abilities as an antioxidant.

Like its relatives dill and fennel, anise is known for its digestive properties, particularly when the seeds are used in extracts or powders. However, there is a good deal of essential oil content found in those seeds that can be distilled for varying and sometimes more targeted uses and benefits of anise oil.

5 Health Benefits of Anise Oil Uses

Now that we know what anise oil is and how to use it safely, why should we use it at all? Here are five benefits of anise oil and uses that are backed by research.

1. ANISE OIL USES – ANTI-INFLAMMATORY PAIN RELIEF

A major constituent of anise seed oil, anethole, was tested in 2014 for its pain-relieving abilities apart from simply making the individual feel sedated. The results were fairly clear that the compound helped to lessen pain without creating sedation, most likely thanks to anti-inflammatory actions.

This backs traditional uses as a pain reliever, particularly as an oil for muscle pain and inflammatory discomfort.

Indications: Massage oil, diluted topical application.

2. ANISE OIL USES – MUSCLE RELAXANT

In a similar vein, anise essential oil appears to relax muscles, which would also contribute to pain relief in many cases. To watch this action take place, researchers tested anise essential oil on pigs to evaluate the tracheal muscles' response to the application. The essential oil showed "significant relaxant effects."

Not only did this study create implications for painful, tense muscles and topical applications, but it also demonstrated a bronchodilator response. In other words, breathing could improve in the case of inflamed or congested airways.

Indications: Topical massage of sore muscles, inhalation during respiratory illness.

3. ANISE OIL USES – ANTIFUNGAL OPTIONS

Topical fungal infections are uncomfortable and difficult to get a handle on, and systemic yeast can be devastating. Essential oils are often effective against fungal problems, sometimes even more so than other options. Anise in various forms, including the essential oil, seems to be effective against multiple kinds of fungi, including the dreaded Candida albicans.

Indications: Diffusion, diluted topical treatments, periodic inclusion of one or two drops in a lipid dilution mixed into a full culinary recipe.

4. ANISE OIL USES – ANTIBACTERIAL POWERHOUSE

Last but not least, of the anise essential oil actions we're highlighting today, antibacterial effects steal the show. Antibacterial essential oils are incredibly useful, from respiratory illnesses to skin treatments or countertop cleaning solutions.

Anise is one of the essential oils with the distinct benefit of being active against bacteria in the mouth. In one study, a decoction of the whole seed was used to demonstrate antibacterial activity. The essential oil will be stronger and, diluted properly, can add to an antimicrobial oral rinse.

With oils that have content like estragole that require a bit of extra attention, synergy can allow you to use a little less of it while actually obtaining more benefits. Synergy is especially important for antimicrobial benefits, and anise demonstrates this perfectly. In a 2008 study, anise essential oil demonstrated increased antibacterial benefits when paired with thyme essential oil, one of the best-loved antimicrobials out there.

5. ANISE OIL USES – NAUSEA RELIEF

If you think back to the last bout of nausea you struggled with, you'll remember sensitivity to smells. The right, or wrong, scent can have a bigger impact during nausea than under normal circumstances.

A 2005 study combined multiple anti-nausea essential oils – anise, fennel, Roman chamomile, and peppermint – to create a soothing blend for patients in hospice care. While it was not their single treatment for nausea, a majority of the patients who used the blend found improved nausea symptoms. As a non-invasive application, we should utilize our bodies' ability to turn something as simple as a scent into a healing tool.

Indications: Personal inhalers, aromatherapy diffusion, on the collar of a shirt.

Anise Essential Oil Interactions

On top of the mild estragole concerns with ingestion, anise essential oil carries interactions with pharmaceutical drugs, as well. Some common interactions include drugs that act on the central nervous system (e.g., diazepam) and blood thinners. Acetaminophen and caffeine may also change in effects when consumed alongside anise essential oil.

Anise may also include phytoestrogen properties, which isn't actually a problem in most instances; just use caution or speak with a physician before use if you are battling an estrogenic cancer.

Always discuss supplements and essential oil use with your doctor, especially if you are on medication, and learn full interactions before beginning to use essential oils internally. Keeping the dose to culinary levels helps to maintain safety, but drug interactions should always be a top concern.

Estragole Essential Oil Content

It's important to note that anise essential oil is a strong source of estragole, which we've discussed with fennel and tarragon essential oils as a concerning compound.

To quickly summarize, estragole itself has been flagged as a toxic compound, potentially causing cancer or creating other kinds of havoc in the body. Two important distinctions should be made, however, before writing off these important substances: 1) we don't consume estragole on its own, and 2) the amounts needed to replicate that risk are almost impossible to achieve.

The absolute safest way to get around the controversial effects of estragole content is to consume only the whole seed, which contains other compounds thought to mitigate the risks, or the essential oil only in very small quantities. Pregnant and nursing women, children, and anyone with a seizure disorder should avoid internal use to be safe.

DIY Anise Oil Uses and Preparations

You can utilize anise for its strongest benefits in a number of ways.

- Careful culinary inclusion of a drop or two properly diluted in lipids and added to a recipe, remembering that less is more with essential oils
- Antimicrobial respiratory inhalation, combined with eucalyptus or cinnamon
- Antimicrobial mouthwash, with cinnamon, myrrh, and peppermint
- Dilution into a carrier oil for a topical muscle-relaxing massage oil
- Whole-herb and occasional essential oil culinary inclusion for digestive wellness

Become familiar with the safe uses of anise, as well as the GC/MS analysis from your essential oil source, which can tell you exactly how much estragole is in your anise essential oil. Then have fun experimenting with the distinctive licorice flavor and scent as you blend it with more familiar essential oils.

Chapter 8
Fight Cancer and Nausea with Cardamom Essential Oil

Joining ancient aromatic spices like cinnamon and myrrh, cardamom is rich in essential oil and shares many of the benefits of these classic, fragrant substances. As a whole spice or an isolated essential oil, cardamom essential oil uses are underutilized options for digestive wellness and antioxidant potential.

Types of Cardamom

The common name "cardamom" can refer to two entirely different plants (and their essential oils). *Elettaria cardamomum* is considered to be true cardamom; while *Amomum subulatum* is "greater" or "black" cardamom. Depending on where you live, you may know all of them as cardamon, as well.

Both types of cardamom have their benefits, and if a specific type is required in the benefits in this overview, we'll note it. Both are from the ginger family, both have similar culinary benefits – though black cardamom isn't as sweet – and both are good choices.

Cardamom essential oils are likely to include 1,8-cineole (also found in eucalyptus), terpenes, and fenchyl alcohol, among other compounds. If you're using a cardamom essential oil for specific benefits, make sure you know which one your essential oil source has provided, based on the Latin name, and whether that's the oil you need.

Historical Cardamom Essential Oil Uses

Cardamom originates in India, and as with most Indian spices, found its way to Rome in heavily utilized trade routes. Through written and archaeological record, we know that cardamom and most other traded spices were used for their fragrance – spiritual practices, perfumery, etc. Even if the essential oil itself wasn't isolated as we are able to do today, it was still enjoyed in whatever ways they could employ.

In the Ayurvedic traditions of India, however, cardamom was used as both a culinary spice and medicinal ingredient. True cardamom was the variety of choice, and the fruit pods were used for digestive wellness, nausea, detoxification, oral health, and respiratory health.

This was, of course, the whole or powdered spice, which does contain the essential oil in small percentages. Many of the health benefits of cardamom extend to both whole spice preparations and essential oil.

Today, as we analyze the specific compounds in essential oils and how they behave in the lab and in the body, we are able to verify some of these actions and apply them in our own health and wellness routines.

Top 5 Cardamom Essential Oil Benefits

Cardamom spice as a regular dietary inclusion will mirror ancient uses, or you can utilize the more targeted benefits of the essential oil. These studies reflect some of the more exciting things we know about cardamom essential oil.

Some of them will be specifically about black cardamom, while most will be for the more common true cardamom. In any case, they all give us a good understanding of how best to use cardamom essential oil in our natural remedies medicine cabinet.

1. CARDAMOM ESSENTIAL OIL USES – ANTIOXIDANT

As a whole spice, cardamom is among the Indian culinary choices that scavenge for free radicals and help the body to detoxify. As an essential oil, black cardamom is especially potent as an antioxidant, with "significant activities in all antioxidant assays," as well as antifungal activity.

Indications: A drop in culinary preparations; topical preparations for antioxidant rejuvenation.

2. CARDAMOM ESSENTIAL OIL USES – GASTROPROTECTIVE

The ginger family is renowned for its digestive benefits, from healing and protective abilities to nausea relief. Like ginger, cardamom essential oil is a good aromatherapy option for nausea, having been evaluated for postoperative nausea with good results. True cardamom in various forms, including essential oil, has been evaluated for its protective effects against ulcers, and found to have "significantly inhibited gastric lesions."

Indications: Inhalation for nausea relief; culinary inclusion for digestive improvement and protection.

3. CARDAMOM ESSENTIAL OIL USES – CHEMOPREVENTIVE

The potential for cancer-preventive effects of essential oils to be used in our everyday lives is exciting and promising for the future. Alongside other potent antioxidants, the essential oil content in cardamom shows anti-tumor potential. As with all essential oils, studies are underway to determine exactly how we can best utilize these benefits to prevent cancer and perhaps treat it. Until that day, we can rest easy knowing that our regular essential oil routines are contributing to overall health.

Indications: Inhalation, topical, and culinary use to access potential chemopreventive properties.

4. CARDAMOM ESSENTIAL OIL USES – ANTIBACTERIAL

Essential oils of the major spices and ginger family are often antibacterial, adding a warm touch to a citrus cleaning spray. In 2007, researchers tested this group of oils for their major components and ability to mitigate the growth of bacteria. Black cardamom in particular was found to "inhibit growth of all tested bacteria," including E. coli, Staph. aureus, and Listeria. The scent of cardamom mixes well with other antibacterial oils, creating the potential for some incredible synergy in fun combinations – including antimicrobial oral rinses.

Indications: Cleaning sprays, well-diluted wound healing blends, oral health blends.

5. CARDAMOM ESSENTIAL OIL USES – ANTISPASMODIC

The category of antispasmodic covers a lot of ground: easing spasms. It can apply to digestive upsets (stomach cramps, diarrhea) and respiratory issues alike (coughing, tickle in the throat). Since we've already covered digestive wellness, we can take a look at a traditional use of cardamom for respiratory wellness. The presence of 1,8-cineole is our first clue, shared with the respiratory poster-oil eucalyptus. Other research has been conducted toward varying kinds of respiratory benefits, including the extract (not essential oil, but sharing some similar properties) easing symptoms of asthma.

Indications: Steam inhalations, personal inhalers, diffusion with an ultrasonic diffuser.

DIY Cardamom Essential Oil Uses and Applications

For digestive health and general wellness promotion, cardamom can be included in meal prep as a simple addition to a healthy lifestyle. Just blend a single drop into sauces and ingredients that call for that spicy, smoky taste, before including the sauce in the full recipe. The lipid will dilute it, and the light inclusion will be both safe and beneficial.

Other applications include:

- Antimicrobial diffusion or sprays, with citrus, frankincense, and myrrh
- Respiratory steam inhalation, with eucalyptus
- Anti-nausea inhalation, with ginger and peppermint
- Bonus: include cardamom in summertime bug/mosquito sprays with lemon eucalyptus

Ancient spices are some of the most richly scented, richly historical essential oils. Bring a touch of the past into your everyday life with the Queen of Spices, cardamom.

Have you used cardamom essential oil?

Chapter 9
Cinnamon Essential Oil for Cancer, Diabetes and More

Warm, spicy, fragrant, powerful, even dangerous? What comes to mind when you think of cinnamon essential oil uses? Even as a potentially sensitizing and irritating oil, we shouldn't make the mistake of avoiding cinnamon altogether. There are many benefits of this classic spice and essential oil.

Cinnamon Essential Oil Uses and Sources

While we know cinnamon as simply sticks, powder, or oil, there is much more to it than a simple cinnamon source. The flavorful "sticks" we know are derived from the inner bark of a *Cinnamomum* tree, of which there are many different varieties. In fact, cassia essential oil comes from a cinnamon tree – *Cinnamomum cassia*. This is a different essential oil though with it's own therapeutic benefits. This chapter is going to discuss cinnamon essential oil uses though and we'll save cassia for a different book.

As always, variety effects composition, and cinnamon essential oil most commonly comes from the *Cinnamomum zeylanicum* tree. From there, either the inner bark or the leaves can be harvested for distillation. This should be indicated as either "cinnamon bark" or "cinnamon leaf" on your bottle of essential oils.

And yep, you guessed it: the bark and leaf oils have their own composition, as well.

- Cinnamon bark essential oil, on the other hand is steam distilled from cinnamon bark, is reddish/ brown in color and contains mostly cinnamaldehyde (63.1-75.7%) and much less eugenol (2.0-13.3%). It's a known sensitizer and irritant.

- Cinnamon leaf essential oil, for example is steam distilled from cinnamon leaves, is yellowish in color and contains high amounts of eugenol (68.6–87.0%) and some cinnamaldehyde (0.6-1.1%). It's not as common a sensitizer as cinnamon bark is, though it's still a known irritant.

Cinnamon leaf is typically more heavily filled with eugenol – used to relieve pain and inflammation and fight bacteria – while the bark is comprised more of cinnamaldehyde – potent as an antioxidant and antidiabetic.

History of Cinnamon Essential Oil Uses

One of the oldest and most beloved spices, cinnamon was prized in ancient times as a costly and decadent substance, usually burned for its aroma. Biblical mentions include cinnamon as a "choice spice" and part of the holy anointing oil of Exodus.

Further east, cinnamon was used in medicinal preparations in the Ayurvedic model of medicine. It was thought to be "warming" and was used as an antimicrobial treatment or protective substance.

Over time, the spice trade waned and culinary preparations became standard, at least in the Western world. The ability to distill essential oils specifically has opened up another avenue of use for us, and extensive research on this ancient spice has confirmed both aromatherapy uses and medicinal whole-spice uses.

Top 5 Cinnamon Essential Oil Uses

Because the leaf and bark oils work differently, I'll note where one is preferred over the other. The safest use for essential oil is aromatic, via sprays and diffusion or inhalation methods. Some internal and topical use can be utilized as well, though, as long as you carefully dilute and use appropriate amounts. With that in mind, here are the top 5 uses for your cinnamon essential oil.

1. CINNAMON OIL BENEFITS: ANTIBACTERIAL STRENGTH

Cinnamon oil is well known as antibacterial, and that is translating to varied uses as researchers begin to think outside of the box. In 2015, a couple of interesting studies were released for uses of cinnamon's antibacterial strength.

The first combined antibiotic doxycycline with isolated components of 3 essential oils, one of which being cinnamon – with all three components (carvacrol, eugenol, cinnamaldehyde) found in both cinnamon leaf and bark oils. The combination had a synergistic effect, which could imply some answers to the problem of antibiotic resistance!

The second addressed an issue on our minds for awhile now, that of oral health with natural products. Cinnamon oil on its own was protective against an array of oral bacterial colonies. The oils didn't contain prominent levels of cinnamaldehyde, indicating a potential preference toward leaf oil.

A much earlier study had confirmed more traditional uses for this antibacterial oil – relieving bacterial respiratory conditions. Of the essential oils tested in 2007, cinnamon and thyme rose to the top as most effective against respiratory infections.

Indications: Diluted into alcohol for mouthrinse blends, cleaners, hand sanitizers, room diffusion, respiratory blends for inhalation.

2. CINNAMON OIL BENEFITS: ANTIDIABETIC POTENTIAL

We know that cinnamon as a whole spice can be used for anti-diabetic purposes, helping to lower fasting blood sugar levels. Further research is diving into the way this works, and some studies have found specific compounds of cinnamon are responsible for the effect – compounds also found in the essential oil.

For example, cinnamaldehyde in animal models has been observed reducing glucose levels and normalizing responses in circulating blood. In 2015, researchers found cinnamic acid to improve glucose tolerance and potentially stimulate insulin production.

These results are promising, and it will be interesting to see how it ultimately plays out. Diabetes affects a large swath of the population, and natural remedies are needed now more than ever.

Indications: One or two drops diluted in a lipid and included in recipes; inhalation or diffusion; whole-spice culinary inclusion.

3. CINNAMON OIL BENEFITS: ANTIFUNGAL SYNERGY

Especially with such a strong and potentially irritating essential oil like cinnamon, blending and dilution are important. Fortunately, the oils seem to work even better that way. A 2013 study demonstrated the effects of synergy on fungal infections, with the lavender and cinnamon blend performing the best.

Incidentally, lavender soothes what cinnamon may irritate! When creating your blends, use small amounts of cinnamon to enhance the other oils in the combination for an overall effective result.

Indications: Topical fungal infections, diffusion and sprays for in-home fungal growth.

4. CINNAMON OIL BENEFITS: GUT HEALTH PROTECTION

Traditional medicinal uses of cinnamon essential oil include protecting the digestive system. The whole spice is still indicated for this purpose, but aspects of the essential oil are finding their way into studies on this topic, as well.

Eugenol, for example, found in the cinnamon leaf oil, was the subject of a study in 2000. It was found to have a protective effect on the mucosal lining against ulcers and lesions. More recently, in 2015, both eugenol and cinnamaldehyde were explored as additives in animal feed for intestinal protection.

Both cinnamon leaf and bark oils could be utilized here, though the leaf is much milder in taste and should contain the eugenol content that is recurring in studies.

Indications: One or two drops diluted into a lipid and added to recipes; whole-spice use in culinary preparations.

5. CINNAMON OIL BENEFITS: CANCER FIGHTING

Last, but certainly not least, is cinnamon essential oil's ability to fight cancer. Eighty studies to date have investigated cinnamaldehyde's ability to inhibit tumor cell proliferation via trigger cancer cell apoptosis ("programmed cell death") and other mechanisms and the research is clear: cancer patients should be encouraged that natural solutions truly do exist!

Cinnamon Essential Oil Uses of Blends and Applications

For all of its known benefits, cinnamon oil is also known as a sensitizer. And keep to 1% max dilution and no more than 2 drops per culinary dish. Remember that oil and water don't mix, so dilution should happen first in a lipid like coconut oil or another carrier oil.

Use cinnamon oil in:

- Cleaners and sprays with clove and citrus
- Respiratory diffusions with eucalyptus and frankincense
- Culinary preparations with sweet orange
- Highly diluted topical treatments with ginger and lavender

Dilution is the key to unlock the many benefits of cinnamon oil!

Chapter 10
Fennel Oil Remedy for Anxiety, Cramps and Indigestion

Fennel oil comes from the flowering herb, which is related to the carrot family of plants. As a digestive health promoting herb, it is in good company with other beneficial herbs like dill and coriander. The seed is most commonly used in culinary preparations, though the fennel essential oil uses can come from the seed or the aerial (above ground) parts of the plant.

Various preparations and applications of fennel have strong and reliable benefits, and safety is a priority with this potent essential oil.

Traditional Fennel Essential Oil Uses

Native to southern Europe, fennel is found in many Mediterranean recipes, much like its closely related dill, caraway, and coriander. Fennel's primary use in whole-herb preparations has been for digestive health. Seeds would be chewed after a meal to improve digestion, and it was included in many recipes for the same reason.

While the seed was the more substantive part of the plant used, the leaves, stem, and flower are highly aromatic. Like anise, fennel has a touch of black licorice scent and flavor that make it uniquely suited for aromatic preparations.

While we have little evidence of fennel being used aromatically throughout history, there's no question that the ancients enjoyed the fennel oil benefits, if only as they walked by their cultivated plants and brushed the leaves, releasing the oil. Today, we can do far more.

5 Fennel Essential Oil Uses for Better Health

Traditional uses of fennel include everything from digestive wellness to anti-inflammatory, pain relief, antioxidants, breast milk production, and more. The primary use would have been with the whole herb, and many believe that the concurrent compounds help deactivate the risks of estragole.

The essential oil has fewer compounds, but choosing an oil that has lower estragole, using it in appropriate concentrations, and sticking to external use can help us access the benefits of fennel without compromising safety. Here are the top five benefits of fennel I'd like to feature.

1. FENNEL ESSENTIAL OIL USES – IMPROVED DIGESTION

Historically, fennel seeds were chewed after meals to improve digestion. More recently, fennel has been used and tested as a remedy for infant colic. It's important to note that the above concerns led to unfortunate and tragic side effects for some of the infants and the study and its methods should not be repeated.

However, we do know that *"Fennel seed oil has been shown to reduce intestinal spasms and increase motility of the small intestine."* For adults with appropriate application, we can translate that knowledge into safe use. Including fennel in recipes and moderate internal applications, as well as including the whole seed into our diets can help maximize the digestive benefits of fennel seeds.

Indications: One drop diluted into lipids and combined into recipes; topical massage oils for stomach aches.

2. FENNEL ESSENTIAL OIL USES – RELIEVED MENSTRUAL CRAMPS

Fennel essential oil's antispasmodic abilities are showcased when used against menstrual cramps and dysmenorrhea. In 2001, researchers tested fennel essential oil on a rat model of menstrual issues and painful cramping. The essential oil was able to reduce both the frequency and intensity of some of the "cramp" contractions.

The soothing actions of aromatherapy are well suited to this kind of application, as each step works together toward the ultimate goal of relief. The soothing aroma, calming effects of massage or breathing deeply, and medicinal actions work together to further the results.

Indications: Topical massage oil blended with balancing herbs for PMS and cramping.

3. FENNEL ESSENTIAL OIL USES – CALMED ANXIETY

A potential benefit of fennel that researchers are in the preliminary stages on is that of anxiety reduction. The researchers used internal applications studied on mice, finding significant and promising anti-anxiety results. As an animal model, preliminary test, and internal use study, this isn't a 1:1 application to real life. However, we can utilize it in our inhaled and topical anxiety and calming blends to seek synergistic and added benefits. In other words: *It can't hurt to try!*

This is especially noteworthy in light of the menstrual cycle benefits just described. Both cramping and anxiety tend to be symptoms of PMS and difficult menstrual cycles, and fennel could help to relieve them.

Indications: Anti-anxiety inhalers, topical or inhaled PMS blends, diffusion during anxious times.

4. FENNEL ESSENTIAL OIL USES – INHIBITED FUNGAL ISSUES

Topical antifungals are a big over-the-counter market, yet not all are effective. Fennel essential oil provides a potential alternative, with excellent antifungal actions. From a 2015 study,

With better antifungal activity than the commonly used antifungal agents and less possibility of inducing drug resistance, fennel seed essential oil could be used as a potential antidermatophytic agent.

Inhibiting fungal growth in the form of athlete's foot or other topical infections, or even just in the home environment, can be difficult. This puts fennel among protective and healing sources for combating fungal issues.

Indications: Diluted into topical applications and foot soaks for antifungal treatments.

5. FENNEL ESSENTIAL OIL USES – BREAST MILK PRODUCTION

A 2014 study published in the Veterinary Medicine Journal evaluated what the research literature had to report about *galactogogues* (substances used to induce, maintain, and increase milk production) in both in humans and animals and found anise and fennel to be the most potent; primarily because of the content of *estragole* in their oils. (More on the potential effects of estragole below...)

In a special section about fennel, the authors of this article state, "The first report of its galactagogue properties was by a Greek botanist Pedanius Dioscorides (40–90 A.D)...It has been used as a galactagogue in humans and no adverse effects have been reported yet... *F. vulgare* has been used as an estrogenic agent for centuries. It has been reported to increase milk secretion, improve the reproductive cyclicity, facilitate birth, and increase libido. It contains E2-like molecules, such as anethole and estragole."

Personally, Mama Z can attest to fennel's ability to stimulate breast milk and so can the dozens of women we've coached from low to normal-to-high milk production throughout the years.

Indications: Applying a highly diluted blend of basil and fennel oil around the breasts into the armpit regions has done wonders for our friends, family and clients.

Unfortunately, there has been little research to prove this and it remains a controversial topic in the essential oil community. Many Aromatherapists believe that au naturel is always best. Meaning this: once baby enters the world and has been checked to make sure that everything is ok, the only things that are needed is skin-on-skin time with Mama, immediate nursing, and nothing else. No oils, no creams, nothing. Just Mama and baby. A connection needs to be made between the two, and a primary component is through the sense of smell; which is profound sensitive from birth.

A Parent's Magazine editorial covers this topic well, and here are some key takeaway from their article.

> • *According to Lise Eliot, Ph.D. the sense of smell starts in the womb as baby can detect odors from the foods you eat and aromas you*

inhale through your amniotic fluid.

- *Subsequently, breastfed babies can even "sniff out" Mom sooner than bottle-fed babies because they are held close to her body more often.*
- *Research actually suggests that, shortly after she arrives, baby can recognize the comforting scent that emanates from their mother's breasts, underarms, and even beauty products because of her keen sense of smell,*

Because of this keen sense of smell, many Aromatherapists passionately recommend that Mamas shouldn't use essential oils or scented body care products for several weeks – if not months – to give baby the time to experience the world and not overload the senses.

To this point, I feel it's important to mention that should put things into proper perspective. Moms across the nation regularly wear deodorant, perfume, use aerosols, burn scented candles and bring their baby to places that are filled with fragrances. It's impossible to avoid artificial or natural fragrances.

In fact, Marcia Levin Pelchat, Ph.D., a sensory psychologist at the Monell Chemical Senses Center, in Philadelphia. suggests exposing baby to a variety of scents, and telling her what she's smelling. Pelchat recommends placing safe household items and objects underneath baby's nose – "just be sure she doesn't inhale or touch irritating spices, such as wasabi, powdered mustard, chili powder, or pepper, any of which can create a burning sensation in the back of her nose."

- Aromatic flavorings and seasonings (vanilla extract, cinnamon, paprika)
- Baby shampoo
- Clean diapers
- Coffee
- Crayons
- Flowers
- Herbs
- Leather shoes
- Ripe fruit

Essential Oil Composition

Fennel essential oil can be derived from the "aerial parts" (above ground stems, leaves, and flowers) or the seeds of the Foeniculum vulgare plant, and the seeds are the primary part used in herbal and culinary preparations. Typically, the seed is what is used for essential oils, as well.

Familiar compounds like alpha-pinene and limonene are found in fennel, but the seeds contain varying – and usually high – amounts of another compound that we don't see as often: estragole.

POTENTIAL EFFECTS OF ESTRAGOLE

Estragole is a phytochemical compound found in essential oils like fennel, tarragon, and basil. Interestingly, experts claim that estragole "is a naturally occurring genotoxic carcinogen with a DNA potency similar to the one of safrole." This has led to much controversy, culminating in official statements by health officials:

"...Exposure to [estragole] resulting from consumption of herbal medicinal products (short time use in adults at recommended posology) does not pose a significant cancer risk. Nevertheless, further studies are needed to define both the nature and implications of the dose- response curve in rats at low levels of exposure to [estragole]. In the meantime exposure of [estragole] to sensitive groups such as young children, pregnant and breastfeeding women should be minimised."

Note on Seizures & Hypertension

A 2011 case report tells the story of a women who, "Although she was under antiepileptic treatment and had well-controlled epilepsy, she developed a typical generalised tonic-clonic seizure and remained unconscious for 45 minutes following ingestion of a number of cakes containing an unknown quantity of fennel essential oil." Because of this, the researchers concluded that, "This reported case recalls the fact that fennel essential oil can induce seizures and that this oil should probably be avoided by patients with epilepsy."

There are several epidemiological reasons why this conclusion is false and is out of the scope of this chapter to cover each one, but I'll leave you with this thought: just because fennel oil was a common ingredient in the cakes that this woman ate, it does not prove that fennel was the cause. This is a classic statistics blunder that many make. "Correlation does not imply causation," because there are countless other variables that not being considered (diet, environmental triggers, medicines, other ingredients, and etc.).

This is also a tough one for me to figure out because there's virtually no research on this. Nonetheless, virtually every blog that I see on the topic states that fennel is contraindicated for epileptics and people prone to seizures.

According to Aromatherapist Lauren Bridges, a mother of an epileptic child, this issue has become convoluted by myths and jumping to conclusions prematurely.

"Long story short, a lot of the seizure lists floating around the internet are not accurate nor real pictures of the risks and threats. None of them seemingly account for species or chemotype, which makes a difference in this matter. As far as a list of oils with convulsant properties, I would check essential oils safety expert Robert Tisserand's work, but with the understanding that this list can no way give a complete risk profile because of the nature of epilepsy an other seizure disorders."

Same message applies to hypertension. According to Tisserand "I believe that there is no case for contraindicating any essential oil in someone with high blood pressure. As well as closely examining the evidence above, I also refer to more recent research, which confirms that the four "Valnet oils" present no risk. The lack of compelling evidence is reason enough to let go of this chimera."

If these are areas of concern for you, please contact your physician before using fennel.

Best Ways to Have Fennel Oil Benefits

Fennel remains an important digestive substance in spite of safety concerns. When used in appropriate aromatherapy doses and for the appropriate circumstance, it remains beneficial.

Remember:

- Seizure disorders are contraindicated
- One drop diluted into a lipid should be plenty for a full culinary recipe
- Safety is established for inhalation, topical use, and small, diluted amounts internally
- Don't exceed or override cautions without a trained and certified aromatherapist

These precautions can be considered for the other estragole-heavy essential oils, including anise and tarragon, so that you can feel confident enjoying their health and wellness benefits. Some of the best ways to include fennel essential oil uses:

- Topical antifungal treatments with anise diluted into a carrier oil for topical treatment
- Bath salts mixed with a topical dilution used periodically as a foot soak
- Topical sprays are also beneficial for applying the treatment without leaving the skin to a moist, fungi-inviting environment
- Relieve PMS cramping and anxiety with a topical massage of anise and clary sage
- Add a drop or two of fennel to full recipes for digestive assistance

Chapter 11
Ginger Oil for Digestive Support and Cancer Prevention

Sip some ginger ale, or have a delicious ginger chew – it'll make your tummy feel better! I hear a mom's voice in my head when I think of the benefits of ginger essential oil. Its soothing effects on the digestive tract have been well known and beloved throughout the world for many generations.

Culinary Ginger

Ginger as we know and love it is the rhizome (part of the root) of the Zingiber officinale plant. At the end of the growing season, the whole plant is dug up and the rhizomes harvested for use. Some can be retained for replanting, which starts the whole process again for another year. Ginger stores well and has a wide range of preparation possibilities, which has helped to establish it as a staple from early in human history. The harvested root can be chopped, grated, dried and powdered, even candied. It's added to both sweet and savory recipes, food and drink alike.

Traditional Uses

Not only has ginger established itself throughout history for its flavor and versatility, but the medicinal benefits of ginger are obvious and well suited to its uses. From the journal *Food and Chemical Toxicology* (linked below), ginger has been used for at least 2500 years, traditionally for gastrointestinal health, including:

- Digestive upset
- Diarrhea
- Nausea

And, in more recent years, the review notes that researchers are finding even more potential benefit, specifically in the aromatic compounds: *Some pungent constituents present in ginger and other zingiberaceous plants have potent antioxidant and anti-inflammatory activities, and some of them exhibit cancer preventive activity in experimental carcinogenesis.* Could ginger as a digestive-aid staple have protected earlier generations from the plague of cancer that we currently face today? Details remain to be seen, but we can certainly take a page from traditional recipes to incorporate more ginger into our daily lives. Include more ginger in your diet by making recipes such as:

- Ginger-seasoned stir fries
- Gingersnaps
- Gingerbread
- Ginger ale
- Ginger beer
- Ginger sauces
- Ginger marinades
- Ginger-seasoned desserts
- Candied ginger

The root is well established as beneficial for digestion, and you will get some amount of the essential oil compound with it, as well. For more direct benefits associated with the "pungent constituents" described above, the essential oil can be used.

Ginger Essential Oil Uses and Composition

The benefits of ginger essential oil is also derived from the so-called ginger root (that's actually a rhizome), via steam distillation. As with any essential oil, the actual compounds will vary based on where and how the plant is grown. Still, some of the most commonly present constituents in ginger essential oil include citral, zingiberene, and camphene, all from the terpene category of chemical compounds.

According to an analysis of ginger essential oil from a 2015 analysis, the compounds in ginger essential oil include free-radical scavenging capabilities and boosting the body's natural antioxidants. Ginger essential oil uses include a spicy scent used in perfumery, inhalation, and culinary preparations.

Top 4 Health Benefits of Ginger Essential Oil

We love to diffuse ginger around Christmas time especially for its spicy, festive scent reminding us of holiday treats. There are some specific benefits of ginger essential oil to keep in mind when choosing oils. Ginger's benefits are primarily digestive, but you may be surprised at just how effective it might be – or what else it might be used for!

1. BENEFITS OF GINGER ESSENTIAL OIL – GASTROPROTECTION

Ginger root has been used as a digestive aid as long as it has been used at all. Of course, the whole root carries many benefits in its various components. The essential oil itself still retains the benefit of being a digestive aid, which is both importance for potency as well as ease of use.

A recent study depicted an example of the protective effects that ginger essential oil – as well as turmeric – can have on ulcers specifically. The study was conducted in a lab on rat stomachs, but the essential oil was shown to reduce oxidative stress and reduce the damage the ulcers inflicted.

Including a couple of drops of ginger essential oil in culinary preparations can quickly get it into the diet and into the stomach for a simple, easy way to pack a healing punch.

2. BENEFITS OF GINGER ESSENTIAL OIL – NAUSEA RELIEF

Probably the most reliable and definitely the easiest remedy to "apply," simply inhaling ginger essential oil is quite effective against nausea. My favorite studies on this effect is that of relief for chemotherapy-induced nausea.

A full review of the effects of aromatherapy on nausea found that, of the studies that have been conducted, *"the inhaled vapor of peppermint or ginger essential oils not only reduced the incidence and severity of nausea and vomiting."* Sixty women with breast cancer volunteered to use ginger essential oils during chemotherapy, and the acute nausea as well as appetite loss and functioning were improved over placebo.

Create an inhaler with some cloth that has a couple of drops of ginger essential oil, or simply open the bottle and sniff for relief of waves of nausea.

3. BENEFITS OF GINGER ESSENTIAL OIL – INFLAMMATION

Some of the anti-inflammatory properties that no doubt aid in digestive wellness seem to also help with muscle pain. A trial using Swedish massage with ginger essential oil in short term and long term treatments found improvement in chronic low back pain, even at disability levels.

Add ginger essential oil to carrier oils to massage into painfully inflamed areas.

4. BENEFITS OF GINGER ESSENTIAL OIL – CANCER PREVENTION

In vitro and the markers of their actions inhibited *in vivo* (in the body!) We don't yet have a proven indication of how to maximize these benefits, but including ginger essential oil in your regular aromatherapeutic use can only help!

Suggested Oils for Blending

Synergy is a major part of aromatherapy, which means oils typically perform better when combined with others. Try ginger with these oils for both scent combinations and effect enhancements.

- Citrus: orange, bergamot, neroli.
- Floral: geranium, rose, ylang ylang.
- Woodsy/Earthy: eucalyptus, frankincense, sandalwood, cedarwood.

Chapter 12
10 Peppermint Essential Oil Uses to Live By

When we talk about peppermint essential oil uses, we aren't talking about mints, gum, or candy canes. Really, it's quite fascinating – in a somewhat sad way – that peppermint is so commonly associated with sweet treats rather than profound medicinal benefits. Aside from lavender, peppermint essential oil uses may be the most varied of all our essential oils. And yet we've limited it to Santa Claus and toothpaste!

Is there any reason at all that we wouldn't stock our cabinets with peppermint essential oil? Our culture is seriously missing out!

History & Composition of Peppermint Essential Oil

Peppermint (*Mentha x peperita*) is a hybrid combination of watermint and spearmint that grows prolifically – in fact, it can take over like a weed. The aerial parts – flowers and leaves – are harvested for essential oil production, which is conducted via steam distillation. At this point, active ingredients typically include menthone at around 20% of the composition and menthol at roughly 40%, though these amounts may naturally vary. To get the most out of your preferred peppermint essential oil uses, choose a quality brand.

Typically, peppermint essential oil is used as an antiemetic (helps to prevent nausea) and antispasmodic (helps to prevent vomiting as well as any other harsh gastrointestinal contractions). It's a soothing digestive aid and beneficial during times of illness.

Historically, peppermint dates back as one of the oldest medicinal herbs used in Europe, an ancient remedy for both Chinese and Japanese cultures, and an Egyptian medicine in at least 1,000 B.C. When, in Greek mythology, Pluto pursued the nymph *Mentha*, he transformed her into an herb (guess which?) so that the generations to come would enjoy her just as well as he. Such a colorful legacy is contained well in this cool, accessible, effective substance.

Peppermint Essential Oil Uses in Literature

Stepping away from Greek literature and into the scientific realm, peppermint is found throughout databases of studies and reviews – even more so when we look at its specific component *menthol*. With hundreds and literally thousands of mentions, scientists are all over this remarkable herb. I don't make promises and guarantees often, but peppermint is almost a sure thing: add it to your daily regimen and your life will never be the same.

Nausea Relief

For example, while we all hope to avoid surgery, sometimes it is a necessary part of life – and a common part of surgery is unpleasant post-operative nausea, to the tune of 1/3rd of surgical patients. In 2012, Clayton State University facilitated tests on peppermint essential oil's effects on this nasty phenomena. Moms who are in recovery from a Caesarean especially do not want to deal with vomiting and nausea on top of the mixed emotions of the joy of birth and pain of surgery, not to mention the time that could be spent bonding with their babies. So, moms were chosen for this study, with 35 respondents discovering "significantly lower" nausea levels with inhaled peppermint compared with standard treatments.

Irritable Bowel Syndrome

The use of essential oils is sometimes underestimated when limited to the connotations of "aromatherapy." Topical and occasionally internal applications are relevant, as well. One drop mixed with one teaspoon of coconut oil, rubbed on the stomach or ingested in a spoon of honey, can calm an upset stomach or indigestion in a snap. This remarkable ability is being broached by researchers, marked by a systematic review of the literature that cover's irritable bowel syndrome (IBS) and peppermint, though this treatment typically requires the use of peppermint encapsulated in enteric-coated capsules.

Nine studies were reviewed, spanning more than seven hundred patients, and the conclusion was clear – taking peppermint essential oil in enteric-coated capsules performs much better than placebo when it comes to pain and symptom management. In their conclusion, *University of Western Ontario* researchers stated that,

"Peppermint essential oil is a safe and effective short-term treatment for IBS. Future studies should assess the long-term efficacy and safety of peppermint essential oil and its efficacy relative to other IBS treatments including antidepressants and antispasmodic drugs."

Bug Repellant

One of my personal favorite benefits of peppermint essential oil is bug repellant – especially since I live in mosquito country!

In a comparison of seven commercial bug repellants, Terminix® ALLCLEAR® Sidekick Mosquito Repeller nearly topped the charts. If you aren't aware, this is an "all-natural" blend that lists cinnamon, eugenol, geranium, peppermint, and lemongrass oils. It was very close to a tie with OFF!®, the chemical-laden, DEET-filled commercial brand.

Although I don't recommend Terminix® ALLCLEAR® because I have little faith in a big name company to use true, pure, therapeutic grade essential oils, the lesson is the same. It underscores the efficiency of essential oils, no matter their quality. And an effective essential oil blend most definitely is preferred to harmful, toxic chemicals or nasty 'skeeter bites!

Top 10 Peppermint Essential Oil Uses

1. **Ease Pain Naturally–** For a natural muscle relaxer or pain reliever, peppermint essential oil is one of the best. Try using it on an aching back, toothache, or tension headache.

2. **Clear Sinuses** – Diffused or inhaled peppermint essential oil usually clears stubborn sinuses and soothes sore throats immediately. As an antitussive, the results may be long lasting and beneficial when you're down with a cold, plagued with a cough, or struggle with bronchitis, asthma, or sinusitis. Use peppermint in a homemade cough drop recipe to capitalize on these benefits.

3. **Relieve Joint Pain** – Peppermint essential oil and lavender oil work well together as a cooling, soothing anti-inflammatory for painful joints.

4. **Cut Cravings** – Slow an out of control appetite by diffusing peppermint before meal times, helping you feel full faster. Alternatively, apply a drop or two on your sinuses or chest to keep the benefits to yourself.

5. **Energize Naturally** – Road trips, long nights studying, or any time you feel that low energy slump, peppermint essential oil is a refreshing, non-toxic pick-me-up to help you wake up and keep going without the toxins loaded into energy drinks.

6. **Freshen Shampoo** -A couple of drops included in your shampoo and conditioner will tingle your scalp and wake your senses. As a bonus, peppermint's antiseptic properties can also help prevent or remove both lice and dandruff.

7. **Ease Cough** – The antitussive effect of peppermint can help ease a persistent cough. Try using it in a diffuser or as part of this homemade cough drop recipe.

8. **Relieve ADHD** – A spritz of peppermint on clothing or a touch on the back of your neck can help to improve concentration and alertness when focus is needed.

9. **Soothe an Itch** – Cooling peppermint and soothing lavender combine again to soothe an itch from bug bites or healing sun burns.

10. **Block Ticks** – Stop ticks from burrowing with a touch of peppermint essential oil. Make sure you remove them by their head to lessen your chances of contracting Lyme disease!

Peppermint Essential Oil Uses: Cautionary Common Sense

Be sure to follow professional recommendations, healthcare provider advice, and common sense when using peppermint essential oil. While it is incredible versatile and relatively gentle, it is still a medicinal-quality substance and should be treated with care. As with all oils, make sure to always dilute with a carrier oil and, as always, listen to your body and the wisdom of those who have used aromatherapy before us: essential oils are best in small doses!

Also, don't consume neat. The University of Maryland Medical Center warns that peppermint essential oil can relax the esophageal sphincter and pose risks for those with reflux. Don't consume neat. Taking one or two drops of peppermint in a gel capsule can remedy this risk relatively easily.

Chapter 13
Ancient Digestive Remedy: Tarragon Essential Oil

Think of a fragrant dish simmering on the stove or baking in the oven – which culinary herbs and spices are you smelling? These are often full of aromatic compounds, the essential oils escaping and making your stomach growl. Tarragon is one such culinary herb with an essential oil element. If you haven't tried tarragon essential oil yet, here's what you need to know.

Tarragon Essential Oil Profile

As a member of one of the largest flowering plant families, *Asteraceae*, tarragon is one of around 500 varieties of the species *Artemisia*. Native to Europe and Asia but thriving in North America, as well, tarragon spans traditional uses as well as modern essential oil isolation.

Tarragon grows in an upright, shrub-like formation with narrow leaves and bright yellow flowers. Much like modern use, traditional preparations of tarragon varied from culinary ingestion to medicinal extracts and preparations.

As one of the main herbs in French cooking, tarragon leaves are flavorful and fragrant. The compounds in them are understood to act as an herbal "bitter," stimulating the digestive system to better process food. This can have many implications, some of which translate into the essential oil compounds.

In fact, it was the aromatic essential oil levels that garnered tarragon attention above its cousins in generations past, and it's the essential oil that stands out today.

Top 4 Tarragon Essential Oil Benefits

The whole herb is still likely the best inclusion for maximum digestive stimulation, but there are some important secondary effects that the essential oil has on digestive wellness, as well. Both topical and moderate internal use can yield big benefits with tarragon essential oil.

1. ANTIBACTERIAL FOOD SAFETY

Often overlooked in antibacterial uses, one group of researchers took the opportunity to test tarragon essential oil's bacteria-fighting ability and test it in real-life application. The study, released in 2012, not only tested tarragon for its chemical properties and effects in the lab (which many studies on many products do) but also tested it in a food preservation environment.

The results told us what we already know traditionally about essential oils: they are enhancers. Tarragon was effective against *E. coli* and *Staph. aureus*, and was even effective in protecting cheese during the study. Confirming both aromatherapeutic traditions of blending and tarragon's contributions to food safety, they concluded:

Thus, it is suggested that tarragon EO be used as a part of a combination with other preservation...and can be applied as a natural preservative in food such as cheese.

In both estragole-safety and effectiveness perspectives, tarragon included as part of the overall recipe can be beneficial, enjoyable, and safe in most cases.

Indications: One to two drops blended into a lipid and added to culinary preparations, especially in combination with other culinary essential oils; cleaning blends for antibacterial surface protection.

2. DIGESTIVE WELLNESS

Tarragon as a whole herb carries many traditional uses for digestive wellness, from antidiabetic effects to lipid metabolism to liver protection and ulcer resistance.

Translating those benefits to the essential oil isn't necessarily direct – many of the studies have centered around water infusions and alcohol extracts. As you begin to experiment with tarragon as a culinary herb, you can utilize a drop or two of the essential oil now and then, as well. Consider inhalation and topical belly massages, as well, to introduce digestive wellness compounds in other ways.

Indications: Use of the whole herb; some inclusion of careful internal use; blends for topical massage or inhalation.

3. PAIN RELIEF

Often hand in hand with gastrointestinal wellness is the relief of gastrointestinal pain, and tarragon was used to relieve both concerns traditionally. A 2013 in vitro trial used an animal model to see just how tarragon essential oil might work to relieve painful conditions.

Pain relief was confirmed, validating yet another traditional use of an herb and its essential oil. While the study wasn't in humans or their typical applications, the effects remain and can be utilized in whichever way is most convenient for you until we know more from direct research.

Indications: Massage oil blends, topical stomach ache blends.

4. ANTI-INFLAMMATORY SWELLING REDUCTION

The major compounds anethole and estragole found in digestive herbs like tarragon, anise, and fennel might have some controversy surrounding them, but they also carry benefits. One group of researchers evaluated the effects of anethole and estragole on swollen paws of mice. Not only did the treatment relieve the swelling, but there weren't any signs of toxicity.

This doesn't tell us to throw caution to the wind, but it does demonstrate a couple of important things about tarragon and the other digestive herbs and essential oils. First, pain relief and gastrointestinal benefits are likely tied to anti-inflammatory actions. And second, toxicity in many cases depends on use. Be smart with your oils and stay safe.

Indications: Massage oil and other topical blends, especially for swelling, sore muscles, and inflammatory illness.

Estragole's Controversial Twist

Before we get into the ways you can use tarragon essential oil, it's important to know what you cannot do. One of the main components of the essential oil content in tarragon is called *estragole*, which can also be indicated as *methyl chavicol* and *chavicol*, among other names.

Reviewing similar cautions for fennel essential oil, you'll find that many whole herbs known for their digestive prowess also have concentrated estragole in their essential oils. The complexities of nature are so intriguing!

The bottom line for estragole safety is to use your essential oil in absolute moderation and wisdom. Ask your supplier for a copy of the GC/MS evaluation to know how much estragole is in that batch of tarragon, and only use it internally if the percentage is low and the dilution high. Russian tarragon, for example tends to be low in estragole. In preparations, one or two drops for an entire meal is more than enough to suffice.

Official safety statements for estragole confirm that moderation is key – toxicity levels were far above anything we'd actually consume – however, a few demographics should minimize use:

- Pregnant or nursing women,
- Children, and
- Individuals with seizure disorders.

With that said, tarragon has stood the test of time, and it seems the essential oil will, as well. Here are some of the reason's tarragon (used safely) isn't going away.

How to Use Tarragon Essential Oil

As more research is conducted, we will undoubtedly learn details that will improve our use. Learning how essential oils like tarragon work in the body, why estragole is concentrated in digestive herbs yet not without its controversial effects, and the best ways to get the most out of an oil will come to light bit by bit, study by study. For now, we can mimic traditional wisdom in light of what we do know. Some suggested tarragon uses include:

- Stomachache topical blend, including oils like lavender
- Culinary essential oil use, with one or two drops per recipe and partner oils like sweet orange
- Topical treatments for antioxidant skin health
- Massage oil inclusion for easing tense, painful muscles
- Whole-herb use, taking advantage of the entire composition of tarragon to mitigate estragole and allow for fewer safety concerns

What are your favorite uses for tarragon essential oil?

Chapter 14
Thyme Essential Oil Healing Power and Practical Uses

A perennial that can bunch up as a bush or creep along a forest floor, thyme is a ground cover, soil nutrient, and "living mulch." Really, thyme essential oil uses are similar medicinally to its botanical presence: it's always there, sturdy and without much fanfare, but accomplishes important things.

To obtain the thyme essential oil benefits, the leaf and flower of *Thymus vulgaris*, or garden thyme, are steam distilled. Named either for its strong, herbaceous fragrance (*thymon* – to fumigate) or its association with bravery (*thumon* – courage) , thyme's "roots" reach back to ancient Greece.

Thyme Essential Oil Benefits: Chemical Properties

Analyzed for its chemical properties, thyme essential oil is comprised of a component called thymol, followed by gamma-terpinine and cymene. Thymol is most studied, with a rash of research covering its food safety and antimicrobial benefits. In fact, it stands out as thyme's most notable function, cleansing of microbes and danger.

Once again, thyme's presence in the botanical world mirrors that of the essential oil realm. As a plant, it grows along the surface of the ground, preventing moisture loss and protecting the soil and the plants around it. As an essential oil, thyme continues it protective mission, cleansing surfaces and the air around it of detrimental microbes and fungal invasions.

The plant world is teeming with these complete packages of nourishment and health! When we fill our homes and lives with naturally protective substances like thyme, along with its fellow nourishing, healing, and relaxing foods, herbs, and essential oils, we add benefits to our whole life – mind, body, and spirit!

I'd be willing to bet that the chemical names and composite structure of an essential oil is probably still not what you're looking for. Unsurprisingly, the technical details rarely hold interest – we want to get right down to the meat of things. What can we DO with the components? For thyme oil, some of the possibilities are pretty promising!

Thyme Essential Oil Uses – 4 Ways Thyme Can Heal

1. THYME ESSENTIAL OIL USES: IMMUNOSTIMULANT

While thyme protects us as an antimicrobial for cleaning and food safety, which we'll look closely at in a moment, it may also help condition us to respond to microbes we encounter. The *International Immunopharmacology* journal published a study in 2014 that demonstrated thymol, a main substance in thyme essential oil, as a white blood cell stimulant and immune-boosting substance. We all talk about health from the inside out, but thyme may be single handedly embodying that philosophy!

2. THYME ESSENTIAL OIL USES – ANTIDEPRESSANT

One avenue that thymol appears to take in the body is through neurotransmitters associated with depression. Published in *Behavioral Brain Research* this year (2015), Chinese researchers followed the effects of thymol on "chronic unpredictable mild stress," observing anti-inflammatory relief on the neurotransmitters that cause depression. Its potential as an antidepressant therapy is exciting and one I'm looking forward to seeing discovered and developed.

3. THYME ESSENTIAL OIL USES – ANTICANCER

In another book, we looked at a study that demonstrated the benefits rose oil carried against acne bacteria. In the same study, cancer cells were also evaluated to see how they could stand up against ten powerful essential oils. Thyme was one of those oils, and it stood out from the crowd as most beneficial against the cells of prostate, lung carcinoma, and breast cancers. While it can't be stated enough that these studies are preliminary, I'm filled with hope for a future where naturally occurring products replace toxic chemicals for cancer treatment and – dare we hope? – cures!

4. THYME ESSENTIAL OIL USES – HORMONE BALANCING

As one of the top herbs for estrogen binding, thyme may be able to help the body balance and regulate hormones. Incidentally, this is not the only time we have seen a potential estrogenic herb noted for its anti-cancer potential, as well. Because cancer frequently holds receptors for estrogen, thus being fed by anything estrogenic, it is often suggested that you should avoid estrogen if you have or are at high risk for cancer. However, this logic should not cause us to avoid essential oils because of potential estrogenic properties.

At this time, there is virtually no evidence suggesting that essential oils are "estrogenic," or that they they contain hormones. Recent studies actually suggest that they do NOT have estrogen-like activity.

Technically, as researchers have put it, "Several aromatic oils have been recommended as phytoestrogens because they include components related to the sex hormones." What this looks like exactly is not clear. But, from what I can tell, using essential oils like thyme can help create homeostasis in the body, which supports proper hormone balance. Essentially, true healing from the inside out – not using essential oils for hormones like you would a drug.

Some Practical Thyme Essential Oil Uses

ANTI-FUNGAL

In a study released this year, thyme joined lemon, basil, geranium, clove, and cinnamon as highly effective against fungi, including *Candida albicans* and the resulting candidiasis. Antifungal properties are important as a cleaning agent, but I'm especially interested in tools to battle systemic Candida struggles. This specific study occurred in vitro (in lab tests), but we have seen other studies demonstrate inhalation as an effective essential oil application against Candida. Diffuse a couple drops each of thyme, cinnamon and clove for a spicy, herbaceous fragrance that can help ward off Candida.

ANTIBACTERIAL

Thyme is an excellent addition to cleaning solutions, with potent antimicrobial properties. To establish antibacterial control in potentially one of the most infections environments – a commercial chicken house – Polish scientists used essential oil mists and monitored the antibacterial results. Both peppermint and thyme mixed with water were tested separately for three days, with both exhibiting strengths against specific bacteria. Combining antimicrobial and antibacterial oils helps to facilitate that incredible synergistic effect that feels like magic – with each oil enhancing the abilities of the other. Diffuse thyme, peppermint, and lemon for an energizing and disinfecting effect. Add to a spritz bottle for topical disinfecting, particularly in the kitchen after handling raw meats and other food safety risks.

FOOD SAFETY

Thyme is especially well utilized when we take advantage of its antimicrobial prowess and improve food safety. Commercial applications are intriguing, with the potential for preservation and packaging to occur with natural substances like thyme oil. But safety in our homes is important, as well.

For example, a chicken marinade using thyme and orange essential oils was able to inhibit *Salmonella*. A 2004 study and 2007 study found similarly beneficial effects against *Listeria* and *E. coli*, respectively. Though we should all be practicing good kitchen hygiene and food safety habits anyway, including thyme oil in food preparations may help to make up for shortcomings commercially – if nothing else, it's a bit of added peace of mind!

Conclusion

Modern medicine is the #1 cause of death worldwide. Included in the long list of reasons why are medical errors, side effects to unnecessary surgeries and (you guessed it) adverse drug reactions.

In fact, adverse drug reactions kill more than 125,000 people in the hospital alone. And those are just the reported numbers! The *Journal of Law, Medicine and Ethics* calls this a "hidden epidemic of side effects" from drugs that have few offsetting benefits.

The Safe Solution

So, what's the solution to the #1 cause of death?

To stay away from unnecessary prescription and over-the-counter drugs and use plant-based medicine. The key to understanding this last sentence is to know what "unnecessary" means in regards to medicine.

Necessary medical interventions save people from death. Necessary medical interventions help people cope with pain and suffering (whether emotional, mental or physical) when nothing else helps. *Necessary medical interventions* are rarely the first line of defense - they are normally a "last resort." *Necessary medical interventions* should be temporary, but this is not the case for most people.

Millions of people are becoming aware that drugs and surgery are generally NOT the best first approach ot to their health issues and are frantically searching for natural options to the harmful medicine that they are taking for their health problems.

One natural solution that keeps coming up is essential oils.

Why?

Simply put, because they work!

If used properly, essential oils are one of the safest, most powerful natural remedies and we have a long history of use to guide us on our journey.

And the best part?

They have virtually no side effects, if you use them the right way!

Essential Oils for Abundant Living

The information that we have covered in this book is a great start to helping you regain control of your gut health. Though, many people are looking for more. More instruction. More guidance. More step-by-step, how-to tutorials.

This is where our 10-part Video Masterclass comes into the picture. As our gift to you, we want to give you an opportunity to watch it for FREE during one of our upcoming global screenings!

More than 400,000 have watched our masterclass so far, and the feedback has been powerful.

Distilling down what takes aromatherapists months and even years to learn, the Essential Oils for Abundant Living Masterclass delivers an easy-to-follow [video] roadmap so you can start to use essential oils in your home with confidence.

Discover how to give your medicine cabinet a makeover and start to use essential oils for abundant living → *Simply go to EssentialOilsForAbundantLiving.com and register today!*

Dr. Z's Essential Oils Club

For someone who wants even more support and information, I recommend joining my Essential Oils Club. In addition to getting access to a private community support group where my wife and I are active, we answer YOUR questions during monthly Q & As. There are also loads of other great benefits like:

- Getting access to my entire eBook and recipe collection
- Being able to watch 22 demo videos of how to make our favorite healing recipes

- Tuning into more than 70 expert interviews
- And so much more!

*To check out my Essential Oils Club, go to **EssentialOilsClub.info**.*

Good Bye

It's been an honor sharing my research with you through this book. I hope that have been inspired and feel more equipped to use essential oils to heal your gut! I look forward to staying in touch.

Many Blessings!
~ Dr. Z

References

Introduction

Vighi, G et al., "Allergy and the Gastrointestinal System," Clinical and Experimental Immunology, 153, suppl. 1 (2008): 3–6. DOI: 10.1111/j.1365-2249.2008.03713.x.

W.P. Bowe and A.C. Logan, "Acne Vulgaris, Probiotics and the Gut-Brain-Skin Axis--Back to the Future?" Gut Pathogens, 3, no. 1. DOI: 10.1186/1757-4749-3-1.

E. Rogier, et al., Secretory antibodies in breast milk promote long-term intestinal homeostasis by regulating the gut microbiota and host gene expression, PNAS, 111, no. 8 (2014): 3074-3079. DOI: 10.1073/pnas.1315792111.

T. Loney, et al., "Not just 'skin deep': psychosocial effects of dermatological-related social anxiety in a sample of acne patients," Journal of Health Psychology, 13, no.1 (2008):13:47–54. DOI: 10.1177/1359105307084311.

E. Uhlenhake et. al., "Acne vulgaris and depression: a retrospective examination," Journal of Cosmetic Dermatology, 9, no. 1 (2010):9:59–63. DOI: 10.1111/j.1473-2165.2010.00478.x.

I. Le Huërou-Luron, S. Blat, G. Boudry, "Breast- v. Formula-Feeding: Impacts on the Digestive Tract and Immediate and Long-term Health Effects," Nutrition Research Reviews, 23, no. 1 (2010): 23-36. DOI: 10.1017/S0954422410000065.

E. Blumgart, Y. Tran, A. Craig, "Social Anxiety Disorder in Adults Who Stutter,"
Depression and Anxiety, 27, no. 7 (2010): 687-92. DOI: 10.1002/da.20657.

P. Robinson, et al., " Acne, anxiety, depression and suicide in teenagers: a cross-sectional survey of New Zealand secondary school students," Journal of Pediatrics and Child Health, 42, no. 12 (2006): 42:793–6. DOI: 10.1111/j.1440-1754.2006.00979.x.

M. Gupta. "Depression and suicidal ideation in dermatology patients with acne, alopecia areata, atopic dermatitis and psoriasis," British Journal of Dermatology,139, no.5 (1998): 139:846–850. DOI: 10.1046/j.1365-2133.1998.02511.x

R. Li, et al., "Breastfeeding and Risk of Infections at 6 Years," Pediatrics, 134, suppl. 1 (2014): S13–S20. DOI: 10.1542/peds.2014-0646D.

S. Karmakar, et al., "Development of Probiotic Candidate in Combination with Essential Oils from Medicinal Plant and Their Effect on Enteric Pathogens: A Review," 2012 (2012):457150. DOI: 10.1155/2012/457150.
A.K.C. Leung and R.S. Sauve, "Breast Is Best for Babies," Journal of the National Medical Association, 97, no. 7 (2005): 1010–1019.
Zenith Global, "7% Growth for $50 Billion Global Infant Nutrition Market," https://www.zenithglobal.com/articles/1355?7%+growth+for+%2450+Billion+global+infant+nutrition+market, accessed 4/5/17.
Centers for Disease Control and Prevention, "Antibiotics Aren't Always the Answer," https://www.cdc.gov/features/getsmart/, accessed 4/5/17.
Centers for Disease Control and Prevention, "Antibiotic/Antimicrobial Resistance," https://www.cdc.gov/drugresistance/, accessed 4/5/17.

Chapter 1

https://www.britannica.com/topic/essential-oil
http://onlinelibrary.wiley.com/doi/10.1002/j.2050-0416.1907.tb02205.x/full
http://naha.org/index.php/explore-aromatherapy/about-aromatherapy/what-is-aromatherapy
https://www.britannica.com/topic/spice-trade
http://broughttolife.sciencemuseum.org.uk/broughttolife/techniques/miasmatheory
https://www.ncbi.nlm.nih.gov/pubmed/25369660

Chapter 2

https://www.ncbi.nlm.nih.gov/pmc/articles/PMC3289865/
https://www.ncbi.nlm.nih.gov/pmc/articles/PMC4428202/
https://www.ncbi.nlm.nih.gov/pubmed/20523108
https://www.ncbi.nlm.nih.gov/pubmed/20129403
https://www.ncbi.nlm.nih.gov/pubmed/15629254
https://www.ncbi.nlm.nih.gov/pubmed/21211559
https://www.ncbi.nlm.nih.gov/pubmed/22585103
https://www.ncbi.nlm.nih.gov/pubmed/18376654
https://www.ncbi.nlm.nih.gov/pubmed/21305631
https://www.ncbi.nlm.nih.gov/pubmed/25212146
https://www.ncbi.nlm.nih.gov/pubmed/20579590
http://bit.ly/2zTL0Kg

Chapter 3

http://naha.org/index.php/explore-aromatherapy/safety/
http://www.atlanticinstitute.com/
https://www.accessdata.fda.gov/scripts/cdrh/cfdocs/cfcfr/CFRSearch.cfm?fr=182.20
http://bit.ly/2yPmaOW
https://www.accessdata.fda.gov/scripts/cdrh/cfdocs/cfcfr/cfrsearch.cfm?fr=501.22
https://www.accessdata.fda.gov/scripts/cdrh/cfdocs/cfcfr/CFRSearch.cfm?CFRPart=182

Chapter 4

http://info.achs.edu/blog/author/dorene-petersen
http://bit.ly/2wJXG4B
https://www.fda.gov/Food/DietarySupplements/UsingDietarySupplements/default.htm
https://www.fda.gov/Food/DietarySupplements/UsingDietarySupplements/ucm109760.htm
https://www.fda.gov/Cosmetics/GuidanceRegulation/LawsRegulations/ucm074201.htm
https://www.fda.gov/Cosmetics/ProductsIngredients/Products/ucm127054.htm
https://www.fda.gov/AboutFDA/Transparency/Basics/ucm195635.htm
https://aromaticstudies.com/can-essential-oils-be-considered-as-dietary-supplements/
http://www.anh-usa.org/dshea/

Chapter 5

http://bit.ly/2yhH5Ji
http://onlinelibrary.wiley.com/doi/10.1046/j.1365-2036.2003.01421.x/full
https://jasbsci.biomedcentral.com/articles/10.1186/s40104-016-0079-7
https://www.ncbi.nlm.nih.gov/pmc/articles/PMC2751457/
http://www.ncbi.nlm.nih.gov/pmc/articles/PMC3099351/
http://www.hindawi.com/journals/grp/2012/457150/

http://www.ncbi.nlm.nih.gov/pubmed/20030464
http://www.ncbi.nlm.nih.gov/pmc/articles/PMC3921083/
http://www.ncbi.nlm.nih.gov/pmc/articles/PMC2583392/
http://www.ncbi.nlm.nih.gov/pubmed/24756059
http://www.ncbi.nlm.nih.gov/pubmed/22784340
http://www.ncbi.nlm.nih.gov/pmc/articles/PMC1500832/
https://www.ncbi.nlm.nih.gov/pmc/articles/PMC2515351/
http://www.ncbi.nlm.nih.gov/pubmed/9430014
http://www.ncbi.nlm.nih.gov/pubmed/24283351
http://www.ncbi.nlm.nih.gov/pubmed/25500493
http://www.ncbi.nlm.nih.gov/pubmed/26293583
http://www.ncbi.nlm.nih.gov/pmc/articles/PMC3990147/
http://bit.ly/2i3RUsi
https://www.ncbi.nlm.nih.gov/pmc/articles/PMC2515351/
http://jn.nutrition.org/content/138/9/1796S.full
http://www.nytimes.com/2013/03/28/opinion/antibiotics-and-the-meat-we-eat.html?_r=2
https://www.health.harvard.edu/newsletter_article/stress-and-the-sensitive-gut
https://www.ncbi.nlm.nih.gov/pubmed/25500493
https://www.ncbi.nlm.nih.gov/pubmed/16298093
https://www.ncbi.nlm.nih.gov/pubmed/9430014
https://www.ncbi.nlm.nih.gov/pubmed/26170621
https://www.ncbi.nlm.nih.gov/pubmed/26434144

Chapter 6

https://www.hindawi.com/journals/grp/2012/457150/abs/
https://www.ncbi.nlm.nih.gov/pubmed/25275341
https://www.ncbi.nlm.nih.gov/pubmed/12818366
http://www.sciencedirect.com/science/article/pii/S1878535212000792

Chapter 7

https://www.ncbi.nlm.nih.gov/pmc/articles/PMC3405664/
https://www.ncbi.nlm.nih.gov/pubmed/17373749
https://www.ncbi.nlm.nih.gov/pubmed/25506382
https://www.ncbi.nlm.nih.gov/pubmed/11137352/

https://www.ncbi.nlm.nih.gov/pubmed/16375827
https://www.ncbi.nlm.nih.gov/pubmed/16935829
https://www.ncbi.nlm.nih.gov/pubmed/18226481
https://www.ncbi.nlm.nih.gov/pubmed/22926042
https://www.ncbi.nlm.nih.gov/pubmed/26619825
https://www.ncbi.nlm.nih.gov/pubmed/13680814
http://bit.ly/2ibu26A
http://bit.ly/2yhMd1O

Chapter 8

https://www.ncbi.nlm.nih.gov/pubmed/25278182
http://archive.allayurveda.com/elaichi-herb.asp
https://www.ncbi.nlm.nih.gov/pubmed/18997285
http://bit.ly/2ymJUZD
https://www.ncbi.nlm.nih.gov/pubmed/22392970
https://www.ncbi.nlm.nih.gov/pubmed/16298093
https://www.ncbi.nlm.nih.gov/pubmed/23886174
https://www.banglajol.info/index.php/BJP/article/view/8133
https://www.ncbi.nlm.nih.gov/pubmed/22242564

Chapter 9

https://www.ncbi.nlm.nih.gov/pubmed/21929331
https://www.ncbi.nlm.nih.gov/pubmed/26631640
https://www.ncbi.nlm.nih.gov/pubmed/26165725
https://www.ncbi.nlm.nih.gov/pubmed/17326042
https://www.ncbi.nlm.nih.gov/pubmed/21480806
https://www.ncbi.nlm.nih.gov/pubmed/17140783
https://www.ncbi.nlm.nih.gov/pubmed/25765836
https://www.hindawi.com/journals/ecam/2013/852049/
https://www.ncbi.nlm.nih.gov/pubmed/10930724
https://www.ncbi.nlm.nih.gov/pubmed/25553481
https://www.ncbi.nlm.nih.gov/pubmed/?term=cinnamaldehyde+cancer

Chapter 10

http://www.sciencedirect.com/science/article/pii/S1878535212000792
https://www.ncbi.nlm.nih.gov/pubmed/22899959
https://www.ncbi.nlm.nih.gov/pubmed/12868253
https://www.ncbi.nlm.nih.gov/pubmed/11448553
https://www.ncbi.nlm.nih.gov/pubmed/25149087
https://www.ncbi.nlm.nih.gov/pubmed/25351709
https://www.hindawi.com/journals/vmi/2014/602894/
http://www.parents.com/baby/development/physical/babies-developing-senses/
https://www.ncbi.nlm.nih.gov/pubmed/20334152
http://bit.ly/2ibu26A
https://www.ncbi.nlm.nih.gov/pubmed/21865126
http://roberttisserand.com/2010/08/can-essential-oils-raise-blood-pressure/

Chapter 11

https://www.ncbi.nlm.nih.gov/pubmed/17175086
https://www.ncbi.nlm.nih.gov/pubmed/26197557
https://www.ncbi.nlm.nih.gov/pubmed/24756059
https://www.ncbi.nlm.nih.gov/pubmed/26051575
https://www.ncbi.nlm.nih.gov/pubmed/24559813
https://www.ncbi.nlm.nih.gov/pubmed/24023002

Chapter 12

https://www.ncbi.nlm.nih.gov/pubmed/19768994
https://www.ncbi.nlm.nih.gov/pubmed/22034523
https://www.ncbi.nlm.nih.gov/pubmed/24100754
https://www.ncbi.nlm.nih.gov/pubmed/23092689
http://www.umm.edu/health/medical/altmed/herb/peppermint

Chapter 13

http://www.academicjournals.org/article/article1390551311_Tak%20et%20al.pdf
https://link.springer.com/article/10.1007/s11094-008-0064-3
https://www.ncbi.nlm.nih.gov/pmc/articles/PMC3391558/
http://discovery.ucl.ac.uk/1352036/
https://www.ncbi.nlm.nih.gov/pubmed/24074293
http://www.if-pan.krakow.pl/pjp/pdf/2012/4_984.pdf
http://webbook.nist.gov/cgi/cbook.cgi?ID=C140670&Mask=4&Type=ANTOINE&Plot=on
http://bit.ly/2ibu26A

Chapter 14

https://www.ncbi.nlm.nih.gov/pmc/articles/PMC4391421/
http://www.sciencedirect.com/science/article/pii/s1567576913004761
http://www.sciencedirect.com/science/article/pii/s0166432815003071
https://www.ncbi.nlm.nih.gov/m/pubmed/20657472/
https://www.ncbi.nlm.nih.gov/pubmed/9492350
http://journals.sagepub.com/doi/abs/10.1177/1091581812472209
https://www.ncbi.nlm.nih.gov/pmc/articles/PMC2529395/
https://academic.oup.com/ps/article/92/11/2834/1602366/The-effectiveness-of-peppermint-and-thyme
http://www.sciencedirect.com/science/article/pii/s0309174007003853

About the Author

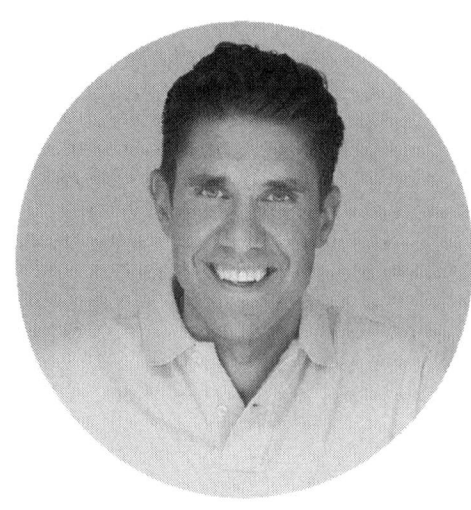

ERIC ZIELINSKI, DC is the author of the national bestseller The Healing Power of Essential Oils. Dr. Z has pioneered natural living and biblical health education since 2003. Trained as an aromatherapist, public health researcher, and chiropractor, Dr. Z started DrEricZ.com (now NaturalLivingFamily.com) in 2014 with his wife, Sabrina Ann, to help people learn how to safely and effectively use natural remedies such as essential oils. Now visited by more than five million natural health seekers every year, NaturalLivingFamily.com has rapidly become the number one online source for biblical health and non-branded essential oils education.

Watch a FREE Screening of My 10-Part Video Masterclass to Transform Your Home (and Life!) with Essential Oils...
Reserve Your Spot Today!
EssentialOilsForAbundantLiving.com

Looking for More?

Join Dr. Z's Essential Oils Club for Monthly Q & A's, Expert Interviews & More!
EssentialOilsClub.info

Other Books By Dr. Z:
The Healing Power of Essential Oils: HealingPowerOfEssentialOils.com
The Essential Oils Diet: EssentialOilsDiet.com